GREEN DRINK DIET RECIPES

THE BEST CLEAN GREEN JUICING RECIPES TO DETOX YOUR BODY NATURALLY

BEST JUICING RECIPES TO DETOX & CLEANSE WITH HEALTHY JUICING FOR WEIGHT LOSS

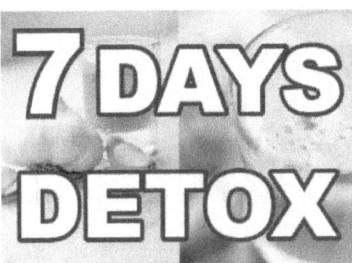

7 DAYS DETOX

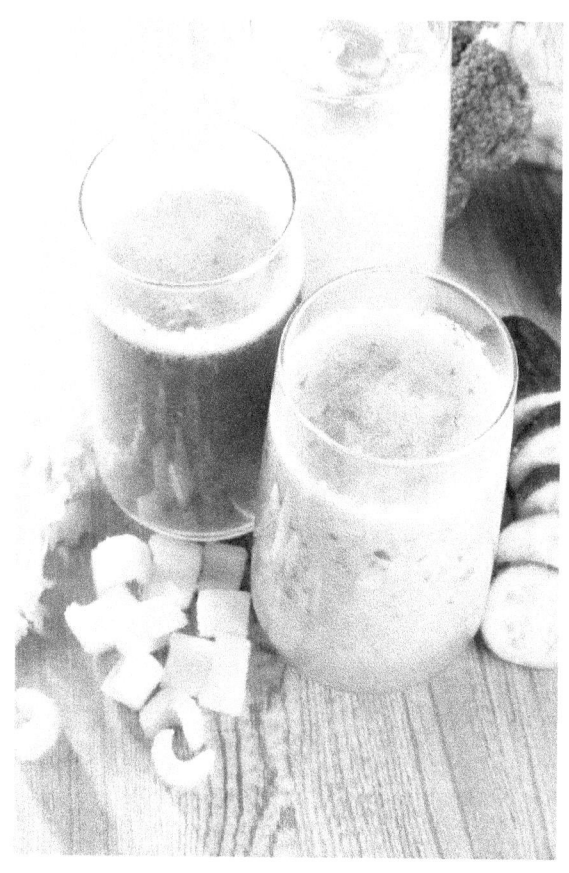

Copyright, Legal Notice and Disclaimer:

have made every reasonable attempt to achieve complete accuracy of the content in this Guide, they assume no responsibility for errors or omissions. Also, you should use this information as you see fit, and at your own risk. Your particular situation may not be exactly suited to the examples illustrated here; in fact, it's likely that they won't be the same, and you should adjust your use of the information and recommendations accordingly.

Any trademarks, service marks, product names or named features are assumed to be the property of their respective owners, and are used only for reference. There is no implied endorsement if we use one of these terms.

Finally, use your head. Nothing in this Guide is intended to replace common sense, legal, medical or other professional advice, and is meant to inform and entertain the reader. So have fun with this complete GREEN DRINK DIET RECIPES guide.

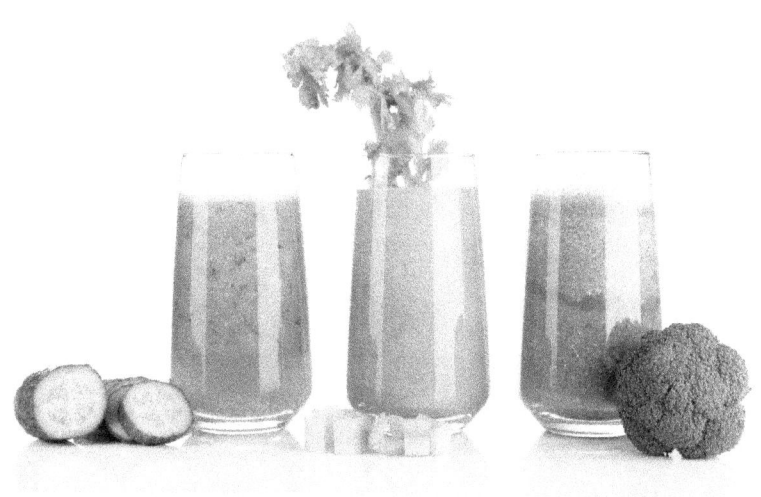

Table of Content

Introduction - Discover What Green Juicing is and why it is good for Your Health – Top Reasons to Consider a Green Juice Detox Diet Now!

Most people have heard about the health benefits of a raw diet and you've maybe learned that a **green juice diet** can promote your wellbeing but you might not be really sure about the real powers of this kind of diet. With this book you will discover all the powers of a green juicing diet and how your body will benefit from consuming these healthy recipes frequently.

This is by far the best and easiest way to introduce veggies into your diet!

The definition of a Green Juice:

A green juice is typically a natural extract made from raw vegetables without any added artificial sugars. Generally it does not contain too many fruits or barely a minimum portion of it. **Most frequently green juices are made from a combination of leafy greens such as**: parsley, kale, spinach, cauliflower, sprouts, broccoli, cilantro, mint, green lettuce, red lettuce, celery, alfalfa, asparagus, basil, baby spinach, carrot tops, dandelion, beetroot leaves, romaine lettuce, Swiss chard, etc…

Some extras can be added to some green juice recipes if desired like zucchini, lemon, lime, fennel or jicama and other natural ingredients further described in this book. You can also add some mild sweet flavor to your healthy recipes by mixing some small amounts of fruits like green apples, kiwi, carrots, beets and others.

Why is it essential to include green juices in your healthy diet?

This is one of the best and most effective ways in which your system is able to absorb tons of minerals, vitamins and enzymes from leafy greens.

Leafy greens hold a wealth of nutrients inside them including:

- They include minerals like: iron, potassium, calcium, and magnesium

- They also include vitamins like: vitamin K, vitamin C, vitamin E, and most of the B vitamins

- They are also rich in **phytonutrients** like: lutein, **antioxidants** like beta-carotene and zeaxanthin, which defend our cells from injury and preserves and promotes the health of our eyes among many other health benefits. Dark green leaves even hold small amounts of Omega-3 fats.

- They are also a great source of natural vegetable protein

- They contain **chlorophyll** and essential enzymes

One surprising thing about green juices is that they actually are very refreshing and they even taste good! You can even add aloe vera juice to some of the healthy juice recipes described in this book for extra healing, nutritional and detox power. **Aloe Vera** has some great healing powers like detoxing your system naturally and improving your digestive system functions as well as being great for your joints. Some wheatgrass can also be added to some of the green juice recipes exposed here to profit from the powers of **chlorophyll** that is rich with nutrients that are very beneficial for your health.

Liquid chlorophyll has amazing health powers for our system; in fact chlorophyll can be referred to as the blood of plants. Its molecular structure almost matches the structure of hemoglobin. Our blood is almost 75% hemoglobin giving this natural liquid extract **the power to boost our energy levels and our overall health when consumed**. This nature´s green liquid blood has the power to regenerate our internal organs, our tissues and our cells by detoxifying our bodies at the same time.

This magical liquid has also the ability to heal internal wounds inside our system, **it improves our blood circulation naturally**; it fights infection and helps to recover our immune system notably and effectively. So this is an essential ingredient that can be mixed with the healthy green juice recipes described in this book. Some additional health powers of this magical nature's potion will be exposed further on in this book as well as the best method to extract this liquid from wheatgrass.

Going green is going alkaline and this can do wonders to your health! **By increasing the amount of chlorophyll that enters your body your overall health and energy levels get a phenomenal natural boost.**

The problem with today´s western societies diet is that there is a proliferation of the consumption of processed foods and unhealthy eating habits like consuming too many red meats, all sorts of fast foods, sugary sodas, excess of alcohol consumption, conspicuous caffeine consumption, saturated fats, dairy products and refined sugars. **This phenomenon intoxicates our bodies creating a hostile and unhealthy environment inside our systems.**

Our bodies were not designed to be processing food machines where you can put anything you want inside without consequences. This is where you should decide which path to follow, the one with the red pill or the one with the green pill. The red pill is all that is associated with processed and unhealthy "foods" that only makes your body sluggish and sick. The green pill is of course all the foods that nature has given us in their raw form as fresh fruits and vegetables and certainly the power of green juices to detox and be healthy.

Every cell inside our systems is affected by the pH level of our internal fluids. If this pH level is extremely acid due to an unhealthy diet then the results are the appearance of different illnesses like cancer, obesity, heart disease, premature aging, fatigue and allergies among many others. Also our muscles and our nervous system are negatively affected when there is excess acid inside our systems. Green juices promote an alkaline healthy environment inside your body. **An alkaline body is a strong healthy body**.

An acidic body is overstressed with toxins introduced by consuming processed foods, a stressful lifestyle, pollution in the environment and it reduces its ability to combat different diseases. An alkaline system is better shield against illnesses like colds and the flu. This is why it is so important to incorporate green juices into your healthy menus.

Green juices are so powerful that they infuse an alkaline environment into your circulatory system. All you need to do is start with a healthy green juice diet like the one described in this book.

There are many reasons of why you should consider green juices as part of your healthy diet, it is not only healthy it is a very satisfying experience. In fact **everybody should give their bodies the opportunity of a healthy cleansing diet like the one provided by green juices**. Here is a list of some of the powers and health benefits your body receives when you consume green juices:

- **With green juicing your system gets all the nutrients it needs on a record speed,** just 15 minutes is the time its gets to those nutrients to be absorbed by your body. With solid foods this takes a lot more time, 5 to 8 hours.

- **With green juicing your body gets the right amounts of calcium and phosphorus** that are essential for your good health and wellbeing.

- **Green juicing is a healthy promoter of a healthy body weight and a slim figure.** It is easier to maintain a toned and slim body when juicing with green juices.

- **Green juicing is an excellent way to introduce into your system all the nutrients that your body needs**. Many times it is just too difficult to commit to the consumption of the daily required dosage of veggies in just one sitting. Ideally we should be eating 5 servings of fruits and vegetables per day according to the USDA (US Department of Agriculture). With green juicing this is easily accomplished and in a very refreshing, easy and healthy way.

- With green juicing **you clear your digestive system and avoid constipation problems** cleansing all toxic material from your colon walls and detoxifying your entire body.

- When you introduce a green juice diet into your system **your energy levels get a powerful natural boost and your entire body will feel invigorated**. These powerful juices contain lots of vitamin A, vitamin B´s, C and D.

- **With green juicing your body gets the protection it needs against inflammation cold** and it is a healthy way to halt the cycle of chronic inflammation that leads to strokes and cardiopulmonary problems. **You entire immune system gets a powerful natural boost**.

- A green juice diet is a great way to be sure that **your cholesterol levels will be under control** and **a healthy way to lower bad cholesterol levels** and triglycerides.

- **With green juicing your skin gets a natural lift and a natural glowing appearance**. Also the elasticity of your skin improves notably thanks to the healing powers of the concentrated nutrients inside the green juice recipes described in this book.

- **The health of your eyes improves notably with a diet based on green healthy juices**. These juices promote a healthy vision and provide important levels of **Lutein** preventing macular degeneration.

- **A green juicing diet gives your body strength due to great amounts of vitamin K contained in these healthy juices**. It promotes a healthy blood circulation preventing the formation of artery clots and heart attacks. This is by a far a better choice than using unhealthy prescription drugs! We have been wrongly accustomed to use prescription harmful chemical based drugs for almost everything when the true healthy response can be found in nature!

- **Drinking green juices is a great natural way to ensure that your digestive system works properly** and effectively by eliminating excess stomach acid and reflux at the same time.

- **When you include these healthy green juices into your healthy menus you also receive all the powers from Omega-3 fatty acids contained in these refreshing beverages**. Omega-3 fatty acids are essential for a good cardiovascular health and they also improve your temper naturally.

- An essential power you get from consuming green juices is that **your body receives tons of antioxidants that shield your cells against free radicals** and oxidative damage.

- Another super important benefit that you obtain when you are on a green juice diet is the **anti-aging powers** acquired through the countless nutrients inside these healthy juices.

One essential tip you must take into consideration when juicing is that you should consume your healthy

refreshing beverages as soon as they are freshly pressed on your juicing machine or mixed in your juice blender. This will ensure that you´ll be getting all the essential nutrients from them since nutrient loss occurs fairly quickly after your juices are in contact with the ambiance.

This is why bottled juices have lost almost all their nutritional value. There is nothing like freshly prepared natural green juices from the comfort of your own home where you know exactly what type of ingredients they are made from.

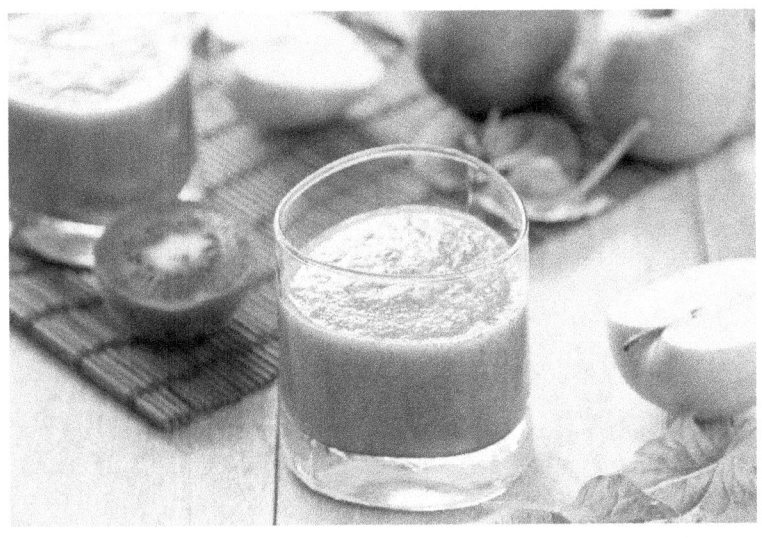

Nature has given us all that we need in order to make our bodies healthier and green juicing is one of the greatest vehicles to achieve this, so start with your green juice diet now!

Best Tips for a Healthy Green Juice Diet

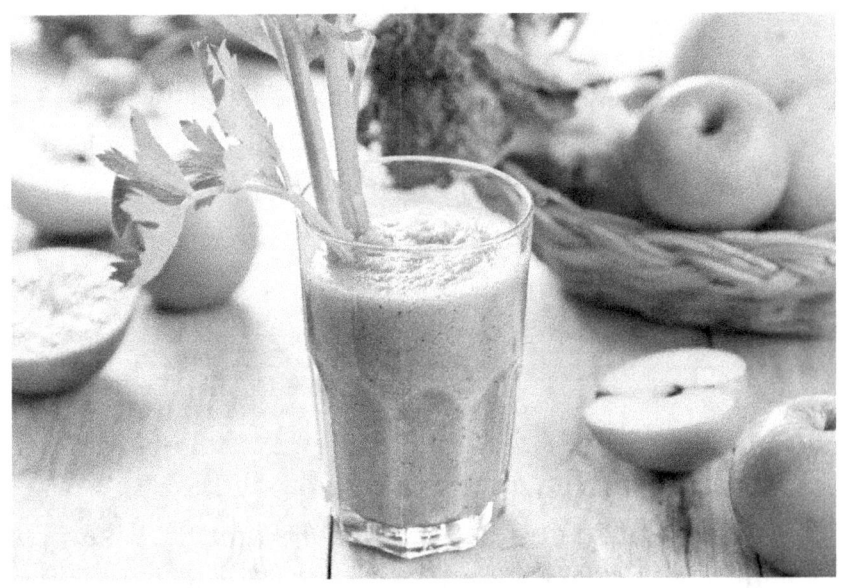

I am sure that you will love green juices once you try them for the first time; this is certainly a great healthy addiction to stick with. But I have to be honest with you this is not love at first sight or better said at first taste. Healthy juices made from raw green vegetables have an unfamiliar and sometimes shocking taste when you first try them. So in a way you will have to train your palate to the new healthy flavors that come from these healthy green juice recipes. This is why I decided to share some tips in order to make this healthy experience much more enjoyable. I can assure you that once you get used to green juicing you will crave form more and more! **Here is a list of some very helpful tips that will help you to get through it with ease**:

- You can add some sweetness to your healthy green juice recipes by adding a sweet fruit like a pear, a banana or an apple or even a carrot. You can also try to add some drops of a healthy sweeter like liquid stevia that has no calories and it is safe for diabetics. This will really help!

- You can dilute your green juices with pure water in order to facilitate the entrance of all these concentrated nutrients into your stomach. When you dilute your healthy juices with pure water you are also softening the raw flavor inherent to all these nutritious natural beverages. You can add some 50% of water to the mix or less depending on your taste; this will make it easier for your stomach to digest all the green components.

- You can improve the flavor of your green juices by adding some vanilla pod to the mix. This not only adds some sweetness to the equation but also a mild sweet scent. One tablespoon of <u>vanilla extract</u> can really turn that raw flavor into something sweeter.

- To make your green juices more palatable you can add some drops of organic lemon juice. This will ease the raw flavor a bit and also increase the detox power of your healthy juices.

- Get a good juicer so your healthy juice recipes won´t lose their healthy nutritional value by overheating problems with the machine. Sometimes some nutrients can be lost due to excess heat caused by a non-professional juicing machine, so if you are serious about juicing my advice is to invest in a good reliable juicer that won´t break or overheat. Centrifugal juicers can do the work sometimes but a heavy duty juicer is better to handle all sorts of greens without breaking. A good <u>low speed juicer</u> works just great!

- Another great tip is to drink your juices slowly and gently savor them in your mouth before swallowing them. This will not only improve your digestion but also will adjust your palate to the new healthy flavors.

- To dilute your juices you can add cucumbers to most of the recipes describe in this book. Cucumbers are low in calories and high in water content making them an ideal ingredient for every green juice. Cucumbers are loaded with nutrients and they contain a substance called **silica** which helps to strengthen your bones and even restore damaged and gray hair to a more youthful state.

- Also keep in mind to consume all your healthy juices at room temperature, the reason for this is that your digestive system is disrupted when you eat cold foods. So a good idea is to leave your vegetables at room temperature at least some hours before juicing.

- Darker leafy greens are richer in nutrients but if you are new to green juicing it is better to start with the least strong juices like the ones with a higher proportion of cucumbers, celery and fennel. Once you get used to green juicing you can start adding other greener and more nutrient rich vegetables like spinach, red leaf lettuce, romaine lettuce, kale, cabbage and green leaf lettuce.

- Always wash your fresh vegetables and fruits thoroughly so you eliminate any traces of pesticides, it is always better to use organic veggies and fruits.

You can use a good natural fruit cleaner to be sure pesticides are effectively removed. A good natural fruit and veggie cleaner is made from 100% natural ingredients and it far more effective than just washing your greens with plain water.

- The ideal is to drink your green juices right away but if you have to store them than use a glass container since plastic containers can leach harmful chemicals. Keep them in the fridge ideally for no more than 24 hours to consume.

- Always clean your juicing machine as soon as you are finished with your juices. Don't let leafy green and wheatgrass pieces accumulate into the moving parts of your juicer.

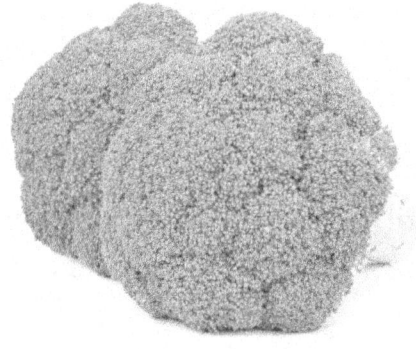

Things to Consider Before Starting a Healthy Green Juice Diet to Detox

It is a good idea to get both a physical and a mental preparation before you start with your healthy green juicing diet. This is an extreme diet to cleanse your body from all toxins that have accumulated inside your system for months if not years so **it is a great idea to prepare your body to receive its much needed healing and cleansing**.

Prepare your body physically for your green juice fast:

It is very important to accustom your body to a softer food regime before making the transition from a solid diet to a liquid green diet. **So the best practice is to eliminate solid foods such as grains, red meats, fish, breads and dairy products at least five days prior to the day you start with your juice fasting diet.** Start consuming more healthy vegetable salads, a lot more fresh organic fruits and vegetables and juices.

Never forget to consume lots of pure water before, during and after your fasting. Raw salads full of greens should be the prelude of your juicing diet. You can also start by replacing some meals with healthy homemade natural juices so your body starts to get used to a more liquid diet. An excellent choice is to replace dinner with a healthy nutritious fruit juice during the week before you start with your green juice regimen.

Start feeding your body with more and more fresh watery fruits like melon and grapes a couple of days before your green liquid diet begins. This will start to detoxify your body while adjusting your digestive system to these new healthy watery nourishments. Your pre-fast diet can also include lots of fresh apples, sprouts, vegetable soups and lettuce.

Starting With a Fast and What You Will Feel:

Please be aware that this is a radical method but a healthy one to detox your system. If this is your first green juice fasting diet it is advisable that you don´t exceed three consecutive days fasting. This is a great way to start eating healthier and to eliminate bad eating habits like the indiscriminate consumption of processed foods and unhealthy fats.

The pH level of your entire system will become more alkaline during your first days of your fasting period. During a short fast lasting a few days, the pH balance of your stomach changes, becoming more alkaline. **You will start to lose weight by eliminating toxins, excess fecal material and parasites**. While all this cleansing process is happening it is likely that you experience some mild headaches, some dizziness and even hunger. A green juice detox diet also has very powerful diuretic properties so you will eliminate more urine than ordinarily.

After a few days of fasting, say by the third or fourth day your liver will start to get rid of toxins polluting your body. This may cause some fatigue, some nausea and even diarrhea since you are on a total liquid green diet. Some skin eruption may even occur during this process. This is a clear signal that your system is detoxifying effectively.

When you extend the period of your fasting diet some other amazing benefits take effect like the **elimination of blood toxins** and the purification of your body organs as well as a deep tissue complete detoxification. This usually happens after a long fasting with green juices, two weeks or more. This means that your entire system is regenerating and you will start to feel younger, stronger and energized. Just keep in mind that **you should start slowly** and then you can go further as your body gets used to a healthier liquid diet. If you are feeling very sick just stop with your fasting and start slowly with solid foods while your system readjusts.

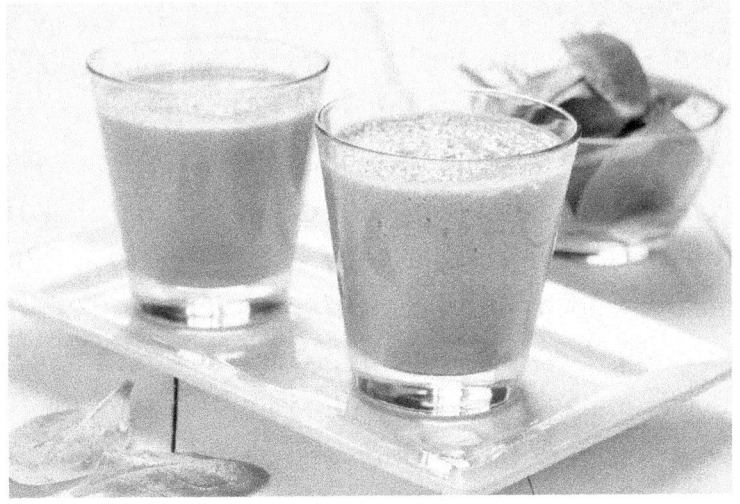

Discover the Best Green Juice Detox Diet Plan

The whole idea with a healthy juicing diet is to replenish your system while at the same type providing your body with essential nourishments found in raw vegetables and fresh organic fruits. **Juicing can be a great natural and healthy method to restore your energy levels and to promote a healthy lifestyle with many added benefits like anti-aging powers.** A comprehensive green juice diet plan does not have to be difficult to implement. The following system of renovation and cleaning will help you not only to detox but also you will relieve your body from stress with natural healing powers.

This plan will create a much needed natural foundation for your system to be healed and purified. The secret behind this natural and healthy method is that **your system will receive an amazing supply of concentrated and unprocessed nourishments in the form of juices made from raw organic fresh vegetables and fresh fruits.** With this type of healthy liquid diet your digestive system will benefit enormously while getting rid of unwanted toxins and excess weight. This is by far the best and most beneficial way of effective fasting.

The first steps you must take to start with this healthy green juice detox diet plan is to eliminate all the poison that is affecting your body and your wellbeing. This has to start by getting rid of alcohol consumption, the elimination of animal meat, no fish, getting rid of animal products like eggs and dairy products, no caffeine, no refined sugars, eliminate wheat and eliminate tobacco at least a week prior to your detox session starts. Ideally your healthy diet before starting with your green juices should be based on the consumption of fresh organic fruits, fresh organic vegetables, beans, vegetables soups and salads.

For this healthy detox plan you should be consuming approximately between 35 and 65 ounces of green juices every day on average. Your main ingredients for this healthy raw liquid detoxifying diet will be spinach, cabbage, celery, beet, carrot, apple, and kale among others.

Please keep in mind that your body will be getting rid of unwanted toxic material trapped inside your system for a long time so you may feel some nausea and some minor headache or sweating. This is completely normal until your body stabilizes and it means that the detox is working. Try to set aside some quiet time while detoxing and ideally create a relaxing ambiance with some relaxing and soothing music.

7 DAY DETOX DIET PLAN

The following juice recipes are designed to make you healthier and to **eliminate toxins from essential vital organs like your liver, your kidneys, your skin, your lungs and your colon**. These juices contain lots of antioxidants, essential nutrients, minerals enzymes and vitamins that will replenish your system internally so you can start looking and feeling much better now!

Day 1: **Super Filler Detox Raw Juice**:

- Two stalks of organic celery
- Two organic green apples
- One organic banana
- 2 organic carrots
- Pure water

All these natural ingredients can be mixed in a blender adding your desired amount of pure water. This is a great detox natural recipe to be enjoyed any time during the day. This healthy juice is great for your kidneys, your colon and your liver.

Day 2: **Delicious Green Spinach Detox Juice**:

- One bunch of organic spinach
- One organic kiwi
- One bunch of organic kale

- One organic banana (to add some sweetness and potassium)
- Pure water

Day 3: <u>**Super Veggie Cleansing Natural Juice:**</u>

- Two stalks of organic celery
- One bunch of organic spinach
- Two garlic cloves
- ½ bunch of organic parsley
- ½ organic onion
- Three organic carrots
- Pure water
- Add some liquid stevia for sweetness

Mix all the ingredients in your bender and add pure water to dilute your green juice as you desire. Spinach is a vegetable loaded with minerals, nutrients and vitamins that contain **flavonoids**, these are very **powerful natural antioxidants** that fight free radicals and cleanse your system effectively.

Day 4: <u>**Super Ginger Detox Booster**</u>:

- One organic ginger root
- 5 organic carrots including tops
- One green organic apple with seeds
- One organic lemon with peel
- Pure water

Ginger is a natural and powerful detox agent. Ginger also stimulates circulation naturally and it is an affective lymph cleanser. This magical ingredient from nature has amazing healing powers like anti-inflammatory properties to naturally heal ulcers, arthritis and colitis. It boosts your immune system naturally and prevents clogged arteries.

Day 5: **Super Potassium Spinach and Parsley Detox Juice**:

- Three stalks of organic celery
- Three organic carrots
- One bunch of organic spinach
- One bunch of organic parsley
- Pure water

Carrots have the natural ability to adjust imbalances in your system. The core of the carrot helps to give strength to your liver which is the most important organ controlling your body detoxification. **Beta-carotene** present in carrots boosts your immune system capacities, improves your digestive system and restores your skin. Carrots are a great natural food to treat acne; beta-carotene helps to heal skin infections causing acne problems and it strengthens your eyes. Natural sugars inside this raw vegetable give green juices a sweet natural flavor. Consuming them also reduces the risk of cancer substantially while getting rid of toxins in the liver naturally and effectively.

Day 6: **Healthy Super Veggie Detox Juice**:

- Three green organic onions including tops
- Two organic carrots

- Two stalks of organic celery
- ½ bunch of parsley
- ½ bunch of spinach
- 6 organic tomatoes
- ½ green organic pepper
- One organic lemon (only the juice)
- Pure water

Mix all the ingredients in your blender with the desired amount of water to obtain a very healthy super veggie detox juice or you can use your juicer. This combination is great to cleanse the liver, your digestive system and to replenish your entire system with healthy nourishments and lots of energy.

Day 7: <u>Super Blood Cleansing and High Blood Pressure Controller Juice</u>:

- One bunch of organic parsley
- Two organic garlic cloves
- 4 organic carrots with tops
- Two stalks of organic celery
- One organic cucumber
- Pure water

Garlic is a natural powerful ingredient containing sulfur that effectively cleanses your liver and your digestive system. It has strong **anti-viral properties** and anti-fungal powers. Combined with these other natural raw elements this is a great healthy detox recipe to heal your entire body and get rid of toxins. A clove of garlic can be added to every one of the above mentioned healthy juice recipes if desired or it can be added in the form of organic garlic powder.

Remember to drink plenty of pure water while detoxifying with these natural juices.

Note: This is not recommended for children, if you are taking prescribed medications, or if you are a person with compromised health i.e. cancer, diabetes or reduced immune functions. Talk to your doctor if you have any doubt before you even attempt to try a detox.

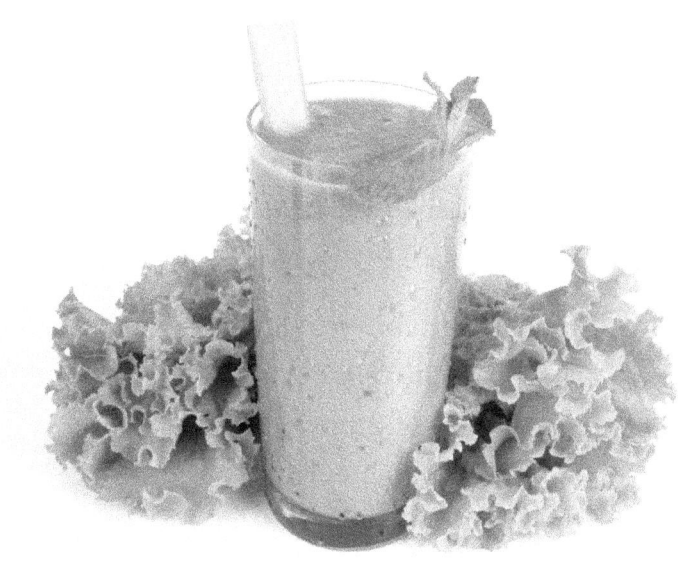

The Differences Between Healthy Natural Juices and Packaged Juice and Why You Need to Stay Away from Those!

Most people tend to think that packaged juices are just as healthy and beneficial as homemade natural juices but unfortunately they are wrong! **Processed industrially made juices are not the safest way to restore your health, period!** The problem with processed juices is that they experience a pasteurization process that affects the nutritional value of these juices.

The process of pasteurization is defined by The American Heritage College Dictionary as "The act or process of heating a beverage or other food, such as milk or beer, to a specific temperature for a specific period of time in order to KILL microorganisms that could cause disease, spoilage, or undesired fermentation."

The problem with this process is that it not only kills bacteria but it also destroys important enzymes and nutrients inherent to raw foods like green juices or

natural fruit juices. There is also a substantial reduction in vitamins with pasteurized or processed juices. Another drawback of these types of processed beverages is that their antioxidant power is greatly reduced due to the exposure of heat in the pasteurization process.

The whole reason for considering a raw juice diet is to precisely profit from all the antioxidant powers, the healing powers and the detoxifying powers that are only present in natural juices not in industrialized processed beverages. These commercial packaged juices are many times presented to the general population as a healthy option but people tend to forget that the majority of them are also loaded with unhealthy refined sugars. Just read the labels and you will find about it. The best option for your health is freshly made green juices that your entire system can really benefit from.

Bottled or Canned Juices vs. Naturally Fresh Prepared Juices

This is an overview of the differences between processed juices and freshly made natural juices using your juice blender or a good juicing machine.

Processed Juices:

- The pasteurization process in bottled juices destroys essential nutrients decreasing the healing powers of these beverages.

- Residues of pesticides may remain inside some of these canned juices and its industrialized manipulation diminishes the enzymes and vitamins. Fruits and vegetables used to produce these juices have been sprayed with multiple pesticides.

- Most of these juices have had many additives and colorants added to their formula to enhance flavor and appearance in an unnatural and unhealthy way. A ton of refined sugar has been added so they "taste better" changing completely their natural flavors and healthy properties. Fruit concentrate is used to produce these juices on a massive scale making them just another sugary artificial beverage disguised in a healthy packaging to make you think it is a healthy option when in fact it isn´t!

- The artificial packaging can also alter the natural flavor of these juices like the ones packaged in metal cans causing a weird unnatural taste. Some of these juices have also been bottled in plastic containers that when exposed to heat or light can leech some chemical residues.

Naturally Fresh Prepared Juices:

Freshly made natural juices are full of enzymes, nutrients, minerals, vitamins healthy fluids, chlorophyll and amino acids that their raw natural ingredients contain.

- Healthy homemade fresh juices stimulate growth and cell repairing
- Natural juices promote healthy blood circulation
- Homemade raw juices promote a healthy digestion and cleanse your body
- These natural freshly made beverages are natural and effective energy boosters
- They are a great alternative to people with malnutrition problems since they provide all the nutrients needed by the human body in a comfortable and easy way to be consumed
- The absorption of nutrients when you consume these natural juices is almost immediate, just 15

minutes after drinking a healthy juice your system receives all the antioxidant powers inside these vegetables and fruits.

- It is a great natural way to effectively treat acne problems.

So always prefer natural juices over processed juices and don´t be fooled by the attractive packaging!

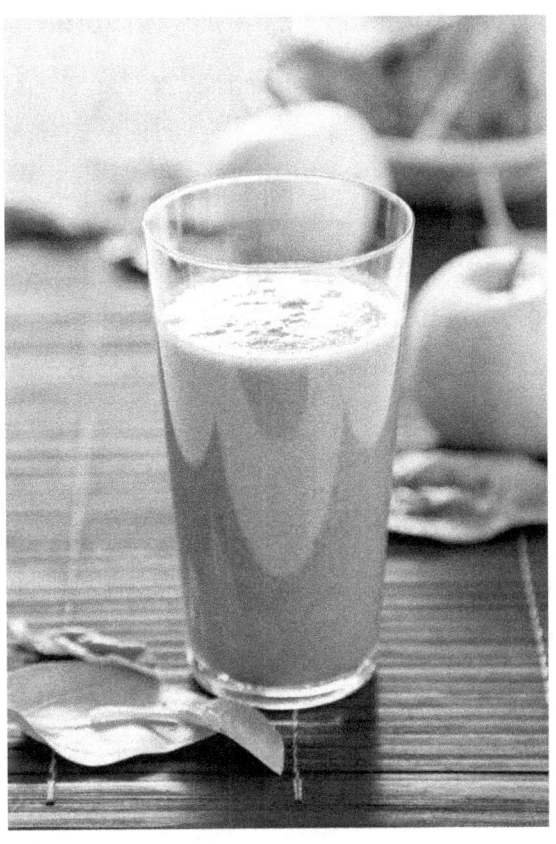

Juicing With Wheatgrass – Discover the Healthy Powers You Get From Juicing With Wheatgrass Juice

Wheatgrass has amazing health benefits and this is why it should be a part of your juicing diet. Like stated before, wheatgrass is a **fabulous and powerful source of chlorophyll, minerals, enzymes and vitamins**. Its similarity with human blood characteristics make this magical liquid a very desirable natural potion to consume for those concerned with their health. So how do we extract this precious liquid to obtain all the powers inside it? It can be extracted with a professional masticating juicer or a much simpler manual wheatgrass juicer.

To start feeling the healthy powers of this powerful nature´s elixir **you can start by drinking an ounce of wheatgrass liquid every day** and then when you get used to it drink two ounces. The idea is to start slowly just as you should do with your green juicing diet to detox. The body needs to adjust but since it is an all-natural ingredient it is only a matter of a few days or a couple of weeks until your palate and your stomach get used to this healthy tonic.

A great tip is to start mixing your wheatgrass liquid extract with some of the healthy green juice recipes described in this book. Even after you are finished with your detox diet plan it is a great idea to keep on juicing with wheatgrass and the best time to do it is one hour before your meals. But undoubtedly **the best time to do it is in the morning on an empty stomach** so you get the most powers this magical elixir contains.

You can drink it straight and pure or if you want you can diluted with distilled water. **Your entire immune system will be restored when you start juicing with wheatgrass.** Some side effects that you may experience when you drink this healthy nature´s tonic are mild nausea and some annoyance over its bitter taste. You can drink some water to dilute this effect. But the benefits of drinking this nature stimulant far exceed the discomfort it causes when you first start with it.

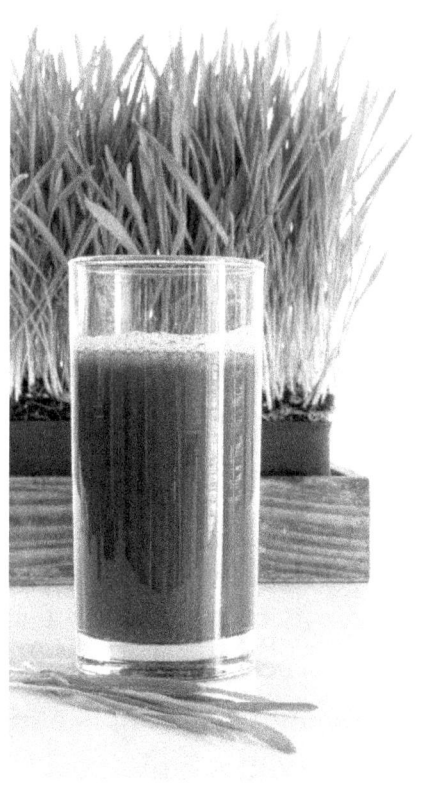

Healthy Powers You Get from Juicing With Wheatgrass Juice:

- **It detoxifies your body naturally**
- It boosts your mental clarity
- **It boosts your energy levels notably**
- It enhances your vision powers
- **It helps to control appetite, this is great for natural weight control**

- It boost your immune system naturally
- **It oxygenates your entire system thanks to its high chlorophyll levels, the chlorophyll molecule is very similar to red blood cells which carry oxygen**
- This healthy juice has plenty of amino acids and numerous vitamins like vitamin C, vitamin E, vitamin K and vitamin B complex that are beneficial for your strength and your health
- **It helps to maintain the alkalinity of your system while fighting acidosis. It is very important to maintain our blood system in balance so you don´t have health issues. Ideally our body internal system should be just above a pH level of 7.0. meaning an alkaline healthy level**
- It has anti-inflammatory powers that are great to heal health problems related to osteoarthritis and rheumatoid arthritis.
- **It has strong anti-cancer powers due to the high amounts of chlorophyll contained in these healthy juices and also thanks the presence of beta-carotene inside wheatgrass. Very strong anti-oxidant properties are present within this healthy elixir from nature**
- This miracle potion has an elevated amount of amino acids that are the building blocks of protein making this healthy juice a great natural source of protein great for building muscle

- **It is excellent to fight anemia problems since it contains high amounts of iron that strengthens your red blood cells while supplying oxygen to your system at the same time**
- It cleanses your lymphatic system and detoxifies your gastro-intestinal system preventing bad breath
- **It effectively and naturally helps to cure wounds, you can actually put some freshly squeezed wheatgrass juice on any wound to see great healing results**
- Consuming this healthy potion helps to effectively remove heavy metals from your system. When consumed frequently it helps to prevent mental illnesses such as Alzheimer´s disease
- **It helps to diminish the damage caused by the environment pollutants such as tobacco smoke and carbon monoxide**
- It helps to cure the itchiness cause by athlete's food thanks to its anti-bacterial powers. You can soak your feet with a mixture of distilled water to get great results
- **It helps to regulate blood sugar levels naturally and effectively making this juice a great alternative for people with diabetes problems**

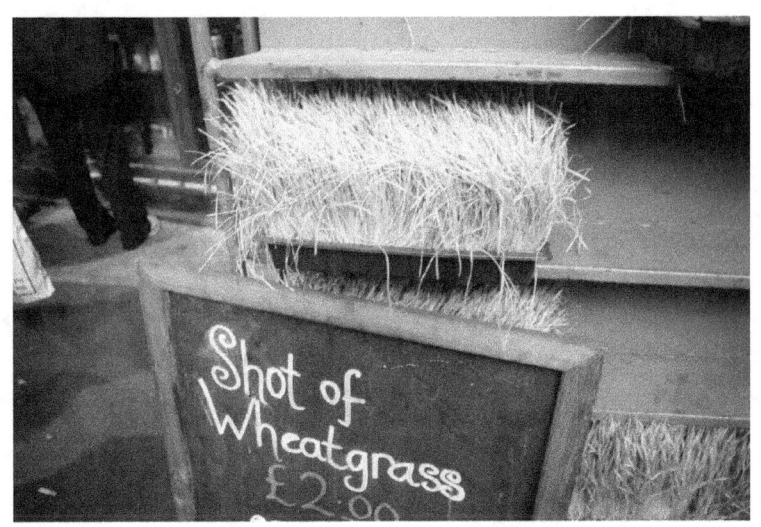

You can even **grow your own wheatgrass** at home:
http://tinyurl.com/wheatgrass-at-home

Discover the Best Vegetables and Fruits to Detox Your Body Now!

Some vegetables and fruits really have strong anti-oxidant powers that make them a great choice to purify our systems internally in a natural and healthy way. Eating fresh organic vegetables and fruits on a regular basis can be used as a natural ongoing detox therapy along with the introduction of green juices into your daily diet.

Our bodies are constantly exposed to countless poisonous substances that pollute our environment and it is essential that we incorporate the right nourishments into our diets so we give strength to our immune system and are able to maintain a healthy alkaline pH. **Always choose organic veggies and fruits and wash them carefully to make sure you eliminate every toxic particle**.

Here is a list of the most powerful vegetables and fruits when it comes to detoxifying powers:

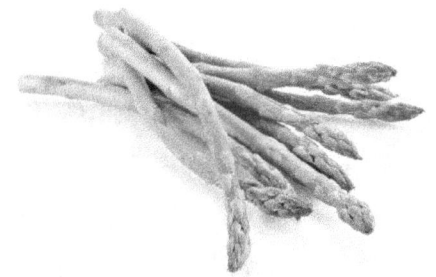

- **Asparagus:** this delicious veggie contains a substance called inulin that promotes your colon health naturally while also improving your digestive system functions at the same time when you eat it or juice it. Consuming this healthy vegetable also encourages the growth of **probiotics**, these are beneficial bacteria that make your colon healthier and balance your intestinal flora.

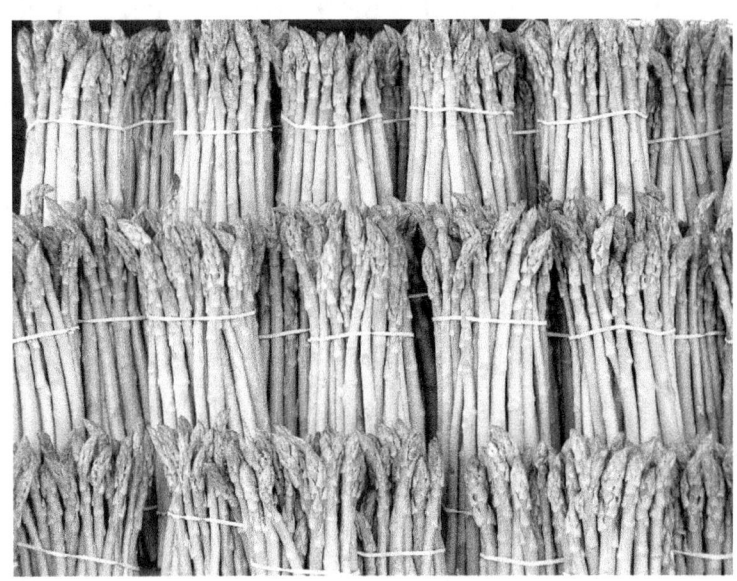

- **Artichokes:** this is a great veggie that supports and enhances the health of your liver and your gallbladder. This powerful leafy green vegetable contains a substance called cynarin that boosts bile production naturally and effectively making it easier to your system to eliminate toxins. The consumption of this yummy veggie also promotes a healthy digestive system and contains dietary fiber which makes it an ideal natural food to maintain a slim figure.

This wonderful green nourishment can be consumed steamed or in the form of juice with some of the healthy green juice recipes exposed in this book. **Eating vegetables along with a green juicing diet is one of the healthiest ways to get a great source of antioxidants**. Don´t overcook your veggies, this way you make sure that nutrients and vitamins inside the vegetables you consume are not lost. High temperature cooking will destroy the majority of those essential components that are good for your health and to detox. So it is a good idea to get a good vegetable steamer to enjoy your solid greens at home.

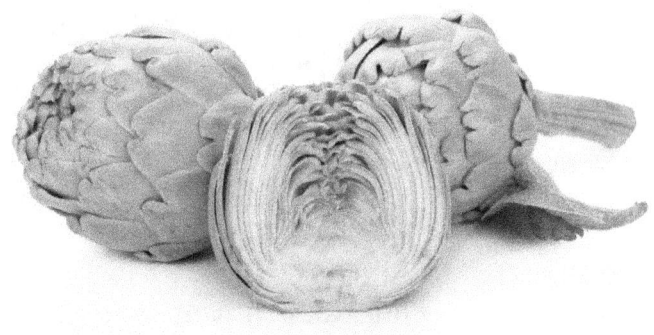

- **Broccoli Sprouts:** this is excellent natural nourishment that has powerful anti-cancer properties. Broccoli sprouts are even more powerful than the mature plant of broccoli. It contains higher concentrations of an **anti-cancer substance called sulforaphane**, almost twenty to fifty times more in fact than mature broccoli heads. According to some serious scientific studies cancer tumors and the appearance of those where substantially reduced in a group of rats that consumed broccoli sprouts. In fact numerous studies have found beneficial results from the frequent consumption of cruciferous vegetables like broccoli containing sulforaphane for cancer prevention and natural cure.

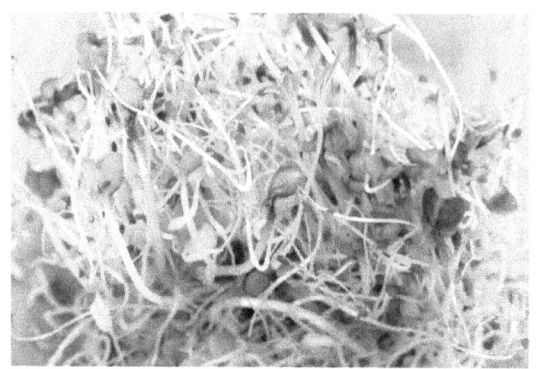

- **Beets:** this is an excellent vegetable to purify your blood. It helps to eliminate alcohol from your blood system and also helps to get rid of processed white flavor and sugars very effectively and naturally. This is an excellent raw leafy vegetable to be juiced and great to detox your body.

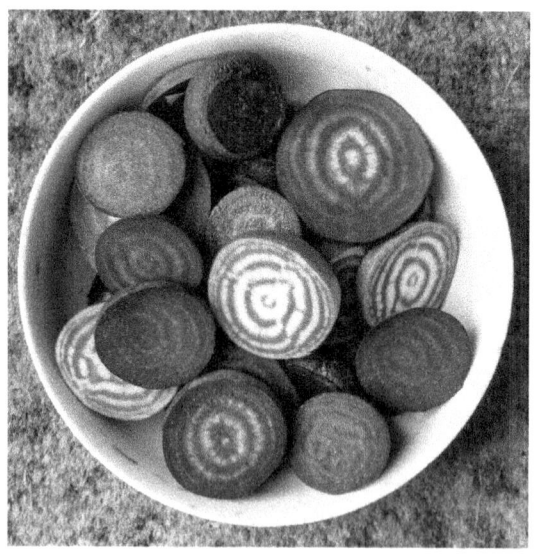

- **Chlorella:** this water-grow micro-algae is excellent to purify your system and to get rid of heavy metals. It is full chlorophyll and tons of vitamins and nutrients that help to cleanse you entire system. It also helps to purify your blood system, cleanses your liver and alkalizes your body. It helps to boost your immune system naturally. It can be taken in the form of <u>natural supplements</u> or in the form of <u>chlorella powder</u>.

- **Mung beans:** this natural nourishment is excellent to absorb harmful toxins from your system naturally and effectively. They are very beneficial for your liver detox.

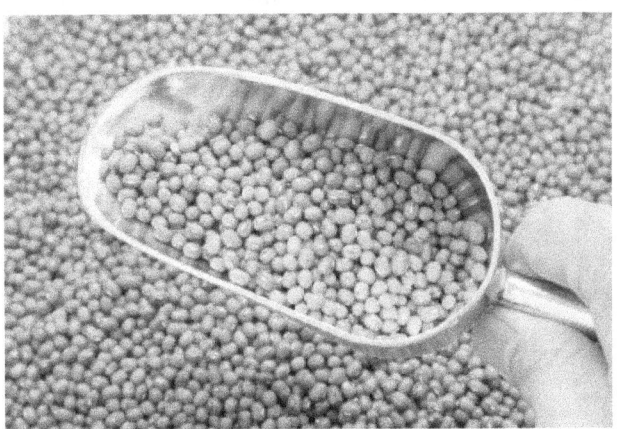

- **Garlic:** this is a great natural detoxifier and a natural antibiotic that helps to cleanse your liver. You can mix garlic cloves with your green juice recipes to get all its detox powers. Adding a clove of garlic to the green juice recipes will just alter the flavor mildly and it is easier to consume this way that by chewing it directly.

Garlic contains allicin and other antioxidant compounds that give this natural nourishment its characteristic tangy flavor. It is rich in minerals like magnesium, iron, zinc, phosphorus, and magnesium and copper making it a natural ingredient to mix with these wonderful detoxifying drinks.

It has excellent antibacterial and has antiseptic powers; large amount of sulfur gives garlic extraordinary medicinal powers. It is excellent for reducing bad cholesterol levels, lowers triglycerides and uric acid and significantly improves circulation thus preventing clots and heart attacks. It also helps regulate blood pressure as it is a natural and very effective vasodilator. When consumed with juices it is easier to digest so you take advantage of all its benefits like the prevention of atherosclerosis by stopping the formation of plaque inside the arteries.

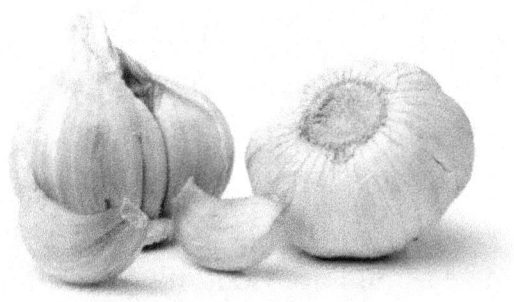

- **Avocado:** although this is technically considered a fruit, this is a great natural green type of food to be consumed when you look to purify your system. It contains omega-3 oils that contribute in the prevention of chronic inflammation by lubricating your intestinal walls at the same time. It also helps your system to get rid of toxins very effectively.

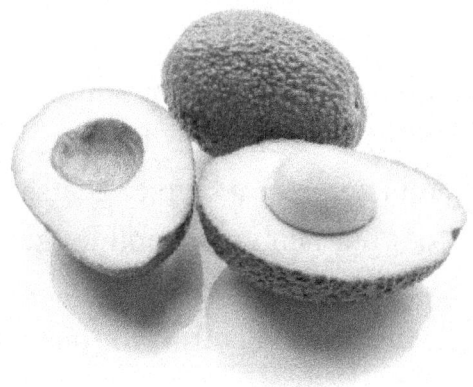

- **Arugula:** this peppery tasty vegetable has wonderful detoxifying properties thanks to the alkaloids it contains. This is a cruciferous vegetable and it belongs to the category of greens that shield your body against different types of cancer. It is filled with anti-oxidants, phytochemicals, minerals and vitamins. These phytochemicals give arugula powerful detoxifying properties and beta-carotene and zeazanthin present in this healthy nourishment act as powerful antioxidants that protect your cells. It is a great green for juicing too.

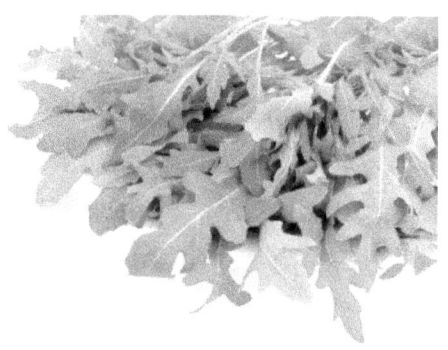

-   **Green Apples:** apples not only are a great natural food full of nourishments but they also have powerful and natural detox agents. Green apples are great for your healthy smoothie recipes; some healthy green juice recipes exposed in this book contain this delicious fruit. In fact you can follow a two day fast just by eating green apples and water to get rid of toxins. This will help your system to get rid of retained water and invigorate your energy levels naturally while clearing your skin.

A substance called **pectin present in apples helps to eliminate heavy metals from your system**. A high level of heavy metals in our bodies makes us age sooner than we should, weakens our immune system and affects our central nervous system. Our polluted environment and some processed foods put these harmful particles into our systems and it is essential to eliminate those from our bodies in a natural way, green apples are just great for that. Another advantage of eating green apples is that they are full of dietary fiber which cleanses your colon helping you getting rid of excess weight naturally.

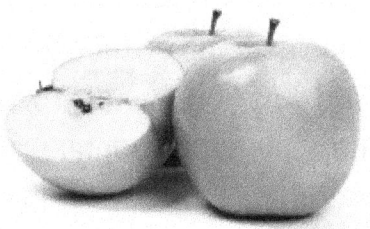

- **Papaya:** this amazing and delicious watery fruits is also great to detox your body thanks to its powerful enzymes. By including this fruit into your diet your digestive system functions improve eliminating toxins and waste material from your colon walls in a natural and effective way. The many nutrients present inside papaya make your skin glow of youth and it is a great fruit to be mixed with some of your green juices as well giving them a sweet natural flavor.

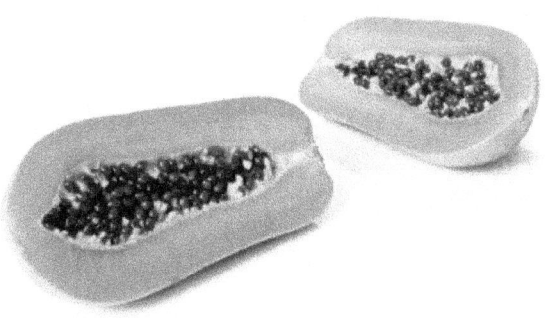

Image courtesy of [FrameAngel] at FreeDigitalPhotos.net

- **Lemon:** this delicious fruit can add some citric flavor to most of your healthy dishes as well as to your healthy juices and contains pectin and soluble dietary fiber that contribute to the natural cleansing of your body.

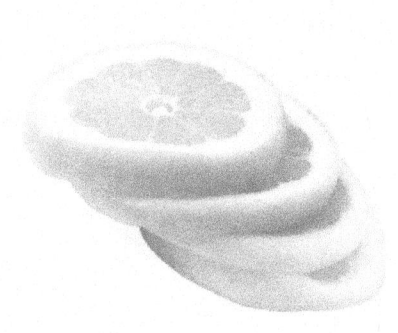

- **Pink Grapefruit:** this is an excellent fruit to eliminate traces of drugs and medicines from your system. It is rich in a substance called lycopene that helps to clear your skin making it look much younger and healthier.

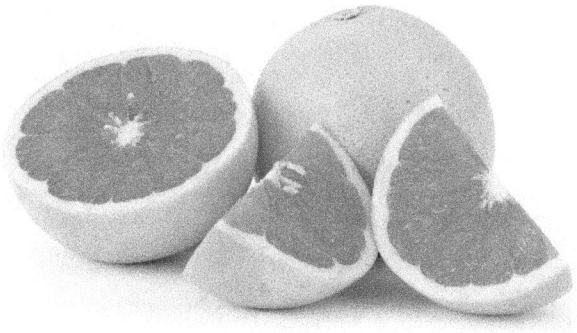

- **Ginger:** the consumption of ginger encourages a healthy blood circulation and promotes a proper and fluid digestion making this another great nourishment to detox your body naturally. It also has strong anti-inflammatory powers. It is also possible to mix ginger into some of the healthy green juice recipes inside this book.

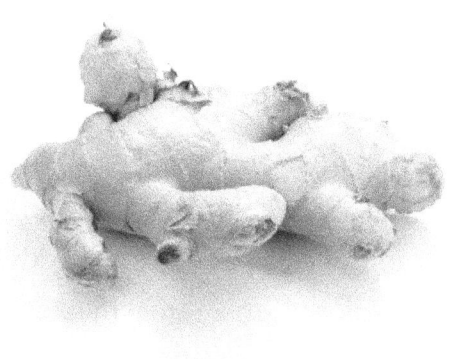

- **Parsley:** this is one of the top sources of chlorophyll and it is a great green to cleanse your liver, your blood and your kidneys. It can be mixed with your foods giving them a natural flavor. Here are some of the powers of parsley: it eliminates water retention from your body, it eliminates bad breath, it is a wonderful antioxidant since it contains flavonoids and vitamin C, it has anti-inflammatory properties and it is good for arthritis conditions. It also contains **beta-carotene** which is another **essential antioxidant** helping to prevent atherosclerosis, colon cancer and diabetes. I can be mixed with healthy salads, soups and obviously with the healthy juice recipes in this book.

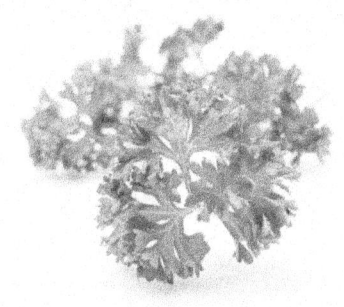

Generally speaking dark leafy greens like kale, spinach, Swiss-chard, cabbage and iceberg lettuce are great to detox since they are rich in essential minerals and have strong alkalinizing properties.

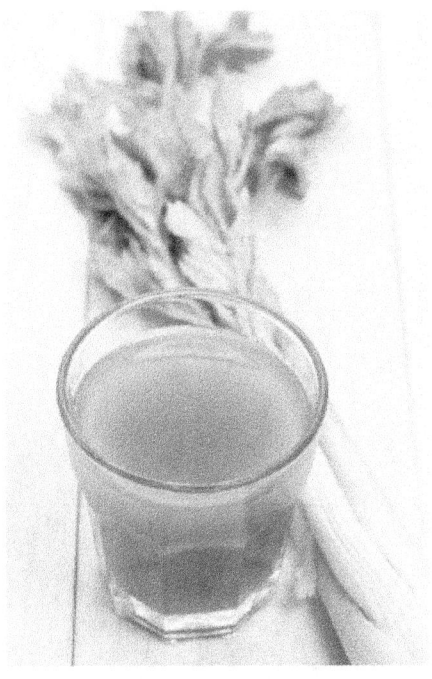

Best Green Juice Recipes to Detox Now!

Super Healthy Spinach Detox Juice:

- One bunch of organic spinach
- One organic cucumber
- One organic kale
- Three organic green apples
- One organic lemon, peeled
- Pure water

All the basic green ingredients are included in this healthy juice recipe. Adding lemon is completely optional if you want a mild citrus taste in your juice. Also by adding lemon or another citric fruit like grapefruit you reduce the green taste a little bit too. All this ingredients can be juiced with your juicer or you can use your juice blender to mix them as well.

Super Healthy Kale and Carrot Green Detox Juice:

- One organic kale
- Two organic carrots
- One organic roman lettuce
- One organic cucumber
- Two organic oranges peeled
- Pure water

- One clove of garlic

You can enjoy this healthy green juice any time during the day and especially at breakfast time to appreciate the citric flavor from oranges.

Super Energizer and Detox Green Juice:

- One organic kale
- A bunch of organic parsley
- Two organic carrots
- One organic beetroot
- One organic cucumber
- Two organic green apples
- One organic lemon peeled
- Pure water

Super Green Veggie Detox Healthy Juice:

- One stalk of organic celery
- One organic cucumber
- Three handfuls of organic spinach
- One handful of organic parsley
- 7 leaves of organic lettuce
- Pure water

Mix all the ingredients in your juice blender or professional juicer. The proportion of water you add to these recipes is completely optional; it all depends on how thick or thin you like your healthy juices.

Super Healthy Spinach and Carrot Detox Juice:

- Three handfuls of organic spinach
- 4 organic carrots including tops
- A handful of organic parsley
- 3 sticks of organic celery
- Pure water

This great mix of veggies provides your system with tons of antioxidant power and powerful cleansing properties. Remember you can always add a little bit of sweetness with some liquid stevia drops.

Super Healthy Parsley Detox Natural Juice:

- Three bunches of or organic parsley (one bunch is approx. 2 oz. or 60 grams) = 1 and 1/2 cups of chopped parsley
- One organic cucumber
- One organic red beet
- 4 organic carrots
- Pure water

Super Green Avocado and Broccoli Detox Juice:

- One avocado
- 2 cups of organic broccoli
- One organic cucumber
- One bunch of parsley
- Pure water

This healthy green juice helps to rejuvenate your skin and it is an excellent source of potassium that improves both your nerve and muscle functions naturally and effectively.

Super Rejuvenating Healthy Asparagus and Carrot Juice:

- Ten organic asparagus spears
- One stalk of organic lemongrass
- Five organic carrots
- One clove of garlic
- Pure water

This healthy juice is **rich in beta-carotene and antioxidants** that will make your skin glow thanks to its numerous vitamins and nutrients. Drink it fresh and enjoy any time during the day!

Super Parsley Detox and Energizing Healthy Juice:

- One handful of organic parsley
- One green organic apple
- Two organic carrots with tops
- One stalk of organic celery
- Pure water

This healthy green juice not only boosts you energy levels thanks to the parsley but it also oxygenates your blood, improves your body odor and cleanses your entire system very effectively. It is full of iron, potassium, magnesium, chlorophyll, cooper and vitamins A and C.

Super Green Broccoli and Celery Healthy Detox Juice:

- 2 cups of organic broccoli
- 3 stalks of organic celery

- One or two cloves of garlic
- One organic tangerine without the peel and with no seeds
- Pure water

This healthy detoxifying juice contains tons of nutrients and minerals like potassium, manganese, phosphorus, copper and magnesium. It is also rich in antioxidants and vitamins like folate, vitamin B1, vitamin B6 and vitamin K.

Super Cucumber and Beet Detox Healthy Juice:

- Two organic cucumbers
- Three organic carrots
- One organic beet
- One bunch of organic parsley
- Two stalks of organic celery
- One organic lemon
- Pure water

You can add a tablespoon of organic garlic powder for extra detox power if desired or one to two cloves of garlic.

Super Healthy Cucumber Detox Juice With Green Apple:

- One organic cucumber
- One green organic apple
- One handful of organic mint
- Grated ginger root
- Two tablespoons of fennel seed

This is a delicious spicy healthy detox juice recipe.

Super Veggie Mix With Broccoli Detox Juice:

- Two cups of organic broccoli
- Three organic carrots
- Two stalks of celery
- One organic beet
- One organic lemon
- Pure water

Broccoli contains very high amounts of healthy antioxidants that help to cleanse your digestive system and your entire body. It is also full of dietary fiber making it an ideal ingredient for your healthy green detox juices. It promotes healthy bowel movements.

Super Body Detox Asparagus and Tomato Juice:

- One organic tomato
- One organic cucumber
- One organic lemon
- One organic asparagus
- Pure water

With this healthy super body cleansing juice you get all the diuretic powers from asparagus that help your system to get rid of accumulated toxins inside and promotes a healthy cleansing of your kidneys as well. Enjoy this healthy juice any time during the day but especially in the morning.

Super Dandelion Liver Detox Healthy Juice:

- One organic cucumber
- Three organic carrots
- One organic peeled lemon
- One handful dandelion
- Pure water

Dandelion is an excellent natural liver cleanser that can be added to any of the recipes described in this book. This herb is also great to improve your circulation naturally and it helps to improve your skin. This herb grows like weed in the fields; you can pick it up directly from there or use it in the form of dandelion root for juicing. Taken in the form of tea it also has some effective cleansing effects on your body.

Super Healthy Skin Detoxifying Juice:

- One stalk of organic celery
- Two organic carrots with tops
- One green organic apple
- Two organic cucumbers
- One clove of organic garlic
- Pure water

Your skin elasticity improves notably with this healthy green juice detox recipe. This healthy watery veggie contains a substance called silica that helps your skin to be more elastic and look fresher.

Super Garden Green Toxin Remover Healthy Juice:

- Four stalks of organic celery
- 8 organic romaine leaves
- One bunch of organic kale
- One bunch of organic spinach
- Two organic green apples
- One bunch of organic parsley
- Grated organic ginger or ginger powder (2 tablespoon)
- One organic lemon
- Pure water

Dark leafy greens like leafy lettuces contain high amounts of chlorophyll and they are a great source of vitamin B complex and silicon. You get a full liver detox with the help of parsley that also stimulates your digestive system enzymes naturally while cleansing your liver, your urinary tract and your kidneys. By adding ginger you give this juice an extra detox power that improves your digestion and also enhances the flavor of this healthy juice recipe.

Super Anti-Aging Cabbage and Carrot Detox Juice:

- 6 organic cabbage leaves
- 6 organic carrots
- Grated ginger or 2 tablespoons of organic ginger powder
- Pure water

This super healthy juice charged with beta-carotene contained inside cabbage makes it the ideal youth potion to drink any time during the day. This juice is also rich in vitamin C and selenium that promotes a healthy skin.

Simple and Effective Green Juice for a Better Skin:

- Two stalks of organic celery
- 4 organic carrots
- One organic green apple
- Pure water

Celery helps to restore the natural moisture of your skin while carrots contribute to a deep internal body cleansing that eliminates toxins in a natural and effective way.

Super Healthy Green Skin Cleanser and Hydrator Detox Juice:

- One organic cucumber
- 7 stalks of organic celery
- One bunch of organic spinach
- One organic green apple
- Pure water

Mix all the ingredients in your juicer or juice blender and enjoy! Celery is an excellent resource of powerful anti-oxidants like vitamin C and foliate. It also contains manganese, potassium, dietary fiber, magnesium, iron, phosphorus and vitamins like vitamin B1, B2, vitamin A and vitamin B6. It contributes to eliminate uric acid from your system promoting the health of your joints and with powerful anti-inflammatory properties. Celery is especially good for your skin since it removes oils and purifies your skin cells naturally removing acne at the same time.

Super Spicy Healthy Detox Diet Juice:

- Six leaves of organic romaine lettuce
- One bunch of organic cilantro
- One organic cucumber
- One clove of organic garlic
- Half organic onion
- One organic lemon
- Half organic jalapeno without the seeds
- Two stalks of organic celery
- Two table spoons of organic ginger powder
- Pure water

This spicy healthy green juice has amazing detox powers and stimulating powers.

Super Green Kale and Onion Detox Healthy Juice:

- three organic kale leaves
- two stalks of organic celery
- three organic carrots
- two organic beets
- one bunch of organic spinach
- half organic cabbage
- half organic onion
- two garlic cloves
- one bunch of organic parsley
- pure water

<u>Super Bitter Gourd Detox Healthy Juice</u>:

- One organic cucumber
- One organic green pepper
- ¼ of bitter gourd
- One organic green apple with no seeds
- One stalk of organic celery
- Pure water

This is a great green juice to be taken first thing in the morning on an empty stomach to detox and flush your system from toxins and waste. As with many of the other green juices it is a matter of time until you get used to the bitter taste but adding apple makes it much more palatable. Remember you can always add a few drops of <u>liquid stevia</u> to sweeten your green juices.

<u>Super Cucumber and Broccoli Detox Healthy Juice</u>:

- Two organic cucumbers
- Two cups of organic broccoli
- Three leaves of organic kale
- One stalk of organic celery
- Two green organic apples
- Grated ginger or one tablespoon of organic ginger powder
- One organic lemon
- Pure water

<u>Super Beet and Green Apple Detox Juice</u>:

- One organic beet
- One organic carrot
- Three organic green apples
- One clove of organic garlic
- Pure water

Super Refreshing Kiwi and Cucumber Detox Juice:

- One organic cucumber
- 7 organic kiwi fruits
- 3 organic green apples
- One piece of organic ginger
- One bunch of organic mint leaves
- Pure water

You can enjoy this very refreshing juice with some ice during any time of the day. You can either use your juicing machine or your blender to mix all the ingredients.

Delicious Avocado and Celery Healthy Juice:

- One avocado
- 4 stalks of organic celery
- One cup of organic broccoli
- Half organic pineapple, cored and peeled
- One organic cucumber
- One tablespoon of ginger powder
- One handful of organic spinach
- One organic green apple
- Pure water

Mix all the ingredients in your juicer or juice blender and enjoy! Although this recipe includes a couple of fruits to give this yummy healthy juice some sweetness it can be considered a green detox juice as well. You not only will enjoy its delicious taste but also all the micronutrients inside this healthy powerful potion. You can drink this yummy juice as a snack anytime during the day even after you are finished with your detox. **Detoxifying your body should be an ongoing culture and the purpose of these healthy recipes is that they serve you as a good guide for your healthy diet from now on.**

Drinking healthy juice recipes like this ones that include avocado help your body to lower bad cholesterol levels naturally and effectively. Avocado contains monounsaturated fats that are good for your hearts health and they help to diminish the level of Triglycerides in a natural way without the use of prescription drugs. Avocados contain also very high amounts of potassium; even more than bananas so there is no need to buy potassium supplements when you include this healthy fruit in your menus and your green juice recipes.

<u>Super Potassium Creamy Green Avocado Smoothie</u>:

- One avocado
- One organic lemon
- Half of an organic banana
- Ice as desired
- Pure water as desired

Mix all the ingredient in your juice blender to obtain a delicious healthy creamy juice supercharged with potassium and healthy nutrients.

Super Green Refreshing Kale and Lemon Detox Juice:

- One handful of organic kale
- Two green organic apples
- One organic lemon
- One clove of garlic
- Pure water

This is a refreshing healthy detox green juice with lots of antioxidant powers.

Super Green Detox Juice With Pineapple:

- Half organic pineapple
- One organic cucumber
- 5 handfuls of organic spinach
- One bunch of organic mint
- Pure water

Super Refreshing Mint and Celery Green Juice:

- Two stalks of organic celery
- Two organic carrots
- Two organic cucumbers
- 6 stalks of fresh organic mint
- 6 stems of parsley
- One tablespoon of ginger powder
- One green organic apple

- Pure water

Super Cleanser Celery and Kale Healthy Juice:

- Four stalks of organic celery
- 7 organic kale leaves
- Two organic green apples
- One piece of organic ginger or two tablespoons of ginger powder
- One organic lemon
- One organic cucumber
- Pure water

You will feel revitalized as soon as you drink this healthy green juice.

Super Healthy Spinach and Green Apple Detox Juice:

- Two handfuls of organic spinach
- Two stalks of organic celery
- One organic cucumber
- One organic green apple
- One organic lemon
- One tablespoon of ginger powder
- Half green organic chard leaf
- One bunch of organic cilantro
- 4 leaves of organic kale
- Pure water

Aloe Vera Detox Cucumber Healthy Juice:

- Two organic cucumbers

- One organic green apple
- Two tbsp. liquid organic Aloe Vera juice
- One tbsp. lemon juice
- Pure water

Aloe Vera has marvelous healing and detoxifying powers for your body.

Delicious Super Cleansing Green Spinach and Parsley Juice:

- One handful of organic spinach
- One handful of organic parsley
- ½ organic pear
- ½ organic green apple
- One small piece of ginger or 1 tbsp. of ginger powder
- One slice of papaya
- One organic cucumber
- Two stalks of organic celery
- Pure water

Super Green Detox Juice With Zucchini:

- Two handfuls of organic spinach
- One organic cucumber
- One organic zucchini
- Two organic pears
- One tablespoon of organic ginger powder

Super Detox Fennel and Mint Juice:

- One bunch of organic mint
- One organic cucumber
- One bulb of fresh fennel
- 4 stalks of organic celery
- One bunch of organic kale
- Pure water

Fennel gives this healthy juice some magic with its crunchy sweet flavor and it is great for reducing inflammation and an excellent source of potassium, folate and vitamin C. You can push all the ingredients through your juicer with the help of your celery sticks or the cucumber if you are using a juicer. Fennel gives your juice a mild licorice aromatic anise flavor.

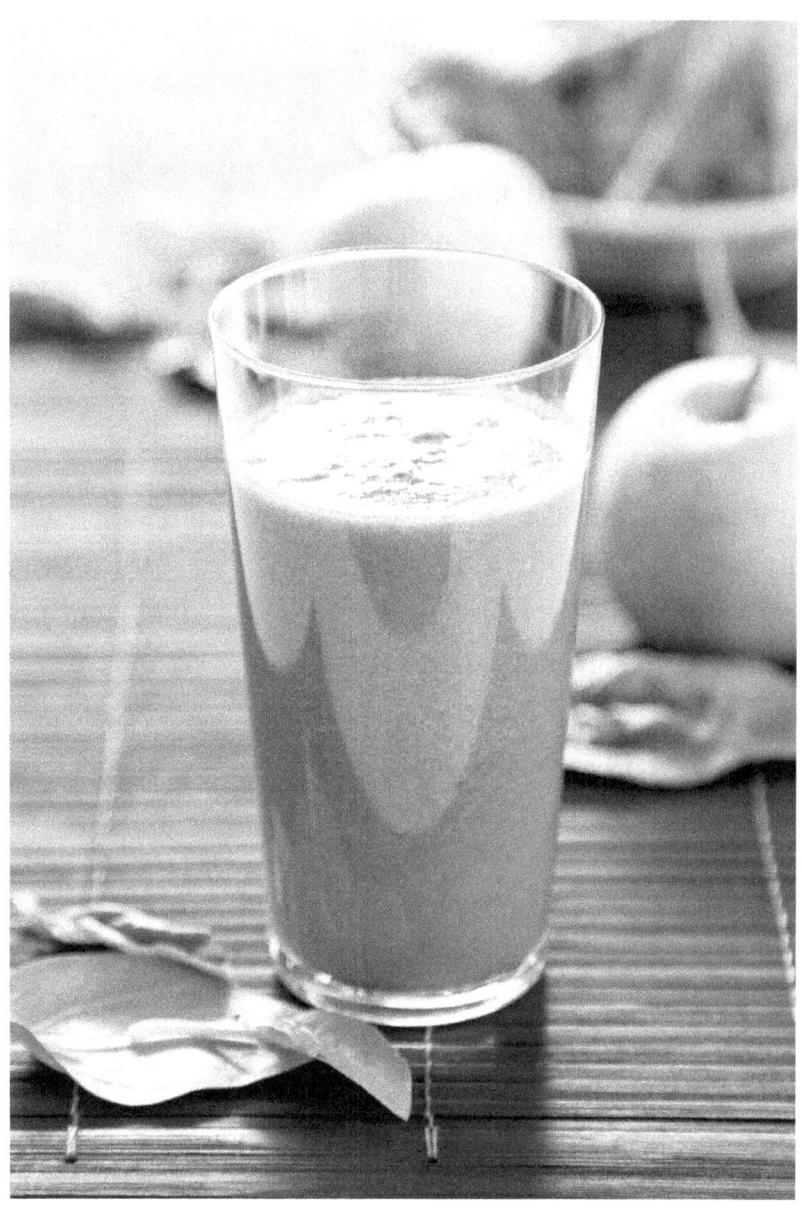

Discover How to Add Some Magic to your Healthy Green Juicing Diet to Detox

You probably already heard about the multiple benefits that Aloe Vera can bring to your skin like the healing powers it has for sunburns, rashes, bruises and cuts. But you may not be aware of the powers of drinking this magic potion and the wonders it can do for your health. This natural tonic contains an incredible number of nutrients, minerals, amino acids and vitamins that make it the ideal companion to be mixed with your healthy green juice recipes.

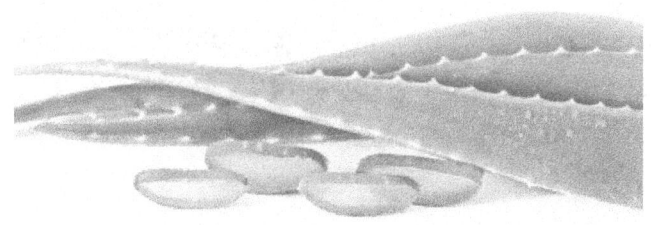

ALOE VERA TO DETOX

Inside this healthy juice you can find amazing healing substances like lectin, mannans, polysaccharides and anthraquinones. All this substances inside the Aloe Vera juice have a wonderful positive health effect on your body. Here is a list of the wonders this natures tonic can do for your wellbeing:

- **Aloe Vera juice is great to detox your body:** the powerful compounds inside this plant help to neutralize toxins. The <u>Aloe Vera juice</u> made from Whole Leaf contains numerous herbal extracts that promote the healthy removal of toxic material trapped inside your body cleansing your liver and your lymph system naturally. It also helps to cleanse you colon walls. It can be used as a natural laxative natural substance that contributes to eliminate heavy metals from your system.

- **It is great for your digestive system**: consuming this healthy nature's potion promotes a healthy functional digestive system since it reduces stomach acid that causes heartburn or acid reflux.

- **It helps to increase your joints elasticity** and it eases inflammation while strengthening joint muscles. Consuming this type of juice is great for people who suffer from arthritis problems. So mixing this healthy liquid natural tonic with your green juices is a great if you want to increase the regenerating powers for your body cell and strengthen aged joints at the same time.

- This healthy potion contributes to **increase your energy levels** in a natural and healthy way. The multiple nutrients found inside Aloe Vera juice give your body the boost it needs to be and stay more active during the day when taken on a regular basis. It is a healthy natural stimulant.

- Consuming this healthy tonic **enhances your immunity system** naturally and effectively. When you introduce Aloe Vera juice into your diet your white blood cells are stimulated so your immune system gets stronger and your body develops the shield it needs to fight diseases naturally.

- It **promotes a healthy weight loss** since it stabilizes your body mass index and stimulates your metabolism naturally. When you consume this healthy juice on a regular basis your system assimilates protein better while boosting your energy levels. Your bad cholesterol levels are also reduced when you make this natural liquid a part of your diet.

- It also **improves blood circulation** in a natural way by improving the capacity of your blood vessels to dilate while regulating your blood pressure simultaneously.

Drinking this juice by itself can sometimes be unpleasant so it is a wonderful idea to use it as another healthy ingredient for your juicing recipes. This is how you add some magic and improved powers to your healthy green liquid diet.

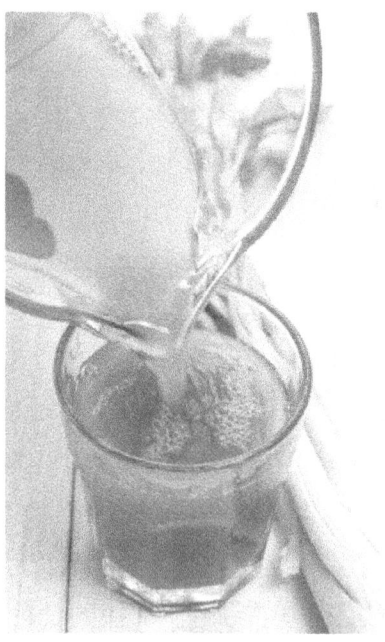

Image courtesy of phasinphoto / FreeDigitalPhotos.net

What to Eat After You Finish With Your Green Juicing Diet to Detox

This is a diet that should be done for a limited period of time. Try not to exceed seven consecutive days on a diet based exclusively on liquids. This is a method of extreme detoxification and it involves making a pause and a post fasting healthy diet. Before you begin with your liquid detox diet, plan the number of days you would be doing it. You don´t necessarily need to stick with it during all 7 days, sometimes 3 or 4 days are enough to eliminate the excess of toxins inside you. It all depends on how healthy you used to eat and what type of lifestyle you had before starting with this detoxifying process.

Try not to stop abruptly with your juice detox diet days; it will require some adjustment for your body to get used to solid foods once again. It is not as easy as ending the detox period and starting to eat cheeseburgers the next day! In fact this is the best opportunity you have to start with a new healthy way of eating from there on. The idea is to reintroduce solid foods into your system slowly and based on healthy nourishments that will not intoxicate your body once again.

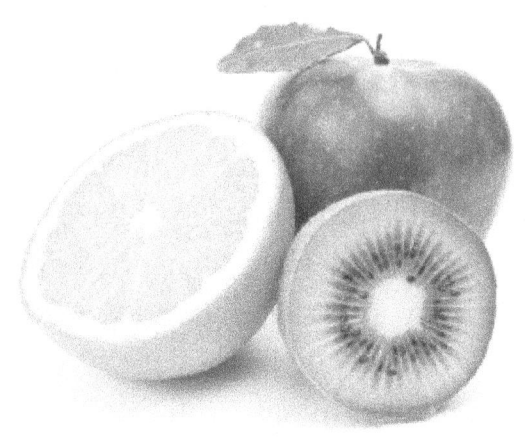

The ideal start after a period of healthy juicing should be based on the consumption of lots of fresh fruits and fresh vegetables. Start with small portions since your stomach size has experience some contraction due to the absence of solid foods during this diet period. **Avoid returning back to your old unhealthy eating habits with excessive processed foods and foods loaded with calories like pizzas, sugary sodas and cakes.** You´ve just made your body an immense good by getting rid of excess weight and toxins so it is not wise to get that back right away.

Control your cravings by eating more fruits and healthy snacks like carrots or celery. You risk of wasting all the efforts done while detoxifying if you don´t start to introduce solid foods gradually into your body. You can feel nausea, weakness or headaches if you start to eat foods that are high in fat or high in processed sugars just after finishing your cleansing period. **The trick is to start slowly so your body doesn't feel a dramatic change in an instant.**

Don't overload your stomach with processed foods once again. Now that your digestive system has had a much deserved break, junk foods are not the best idea to start eating. Every time you feel hungry or a sudden craving attack just grab a fruit and eat it or continue to make these healthy green juices a part of your daily menu.

Never break your detox period by eating junk foods or processed foods; you just have to keep on going until you see the results you want. Interrupting your detox diet like that will destroy the entire process and purpose of the green cleansing liquid diet. You can start introducing different types of salads into your menus after you finish. Your digestive system have been at rest for a period of time and a sudden overload of food will cause you stomach cramps and even nausea and indigestion.

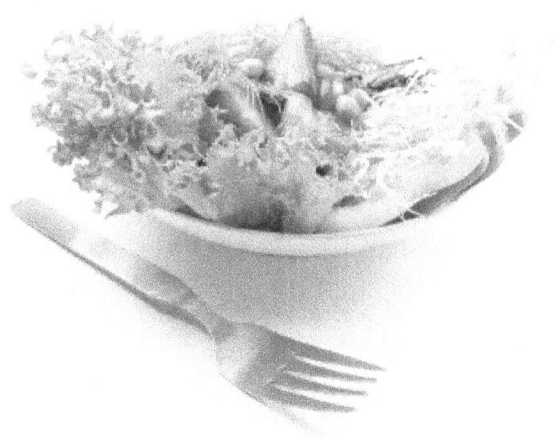

A healthy diet rich in raw foods will improve the entire detoxifying process after you have finish with it. **Consume small portions of fresh vegetables and fruits for the first seven days after cleansing with green juices.** This will support your digestive system recovery and will help it to become dynamic once again in a suave way. The first days you should start with some fresh fruits in the morning and some healthy vegetable salads and soups for lunch and dinner. You can even continue taking some of the healthy green juice recipes you took while you were cleansing your body as they can replace one or more meals. **Returning to solids should be gradual like stated before**.

Slowly you can also start to consume some cereals and grains and try to maintain a healthier diet from there on. By the second week you can start eating more proteins like salmon and lean meats in combination with salads and lots of fresh pure water to keep your digestive system hydrated and clean. Nuts and seeds should be among your first solids after the detox period along with your fruits. Eat them in small amounts.

Discover How to Pick the Right Juicing Machine

You can literally find a myriad of juicing machines and juice extractor brands today in the market. Each one of these brands have different prices and different features that make the task of choosing the right juicing machine a difficult one and sometimes a confusing election. With so many brands and models out there it is important to take into consideration some important factors before making your decision to purchase the right juicing machine.

One of the first questions that have to be resolved when considering your purchase is to know the type of use you want to give to this new machine and what type of juices you want to make. Keep in mind that certain juicing machines are not suited to process wheatgrass, though they may be perfect for handling fresh vegetables and fresh fruits. If you prefer to enjoy the health benefits of wheatgrass juice then a centrifugal-ejection juicer may be a good choice. The best models of this type of juicers feature a powerful motor that handles the task of juicing in less time than a traditional non heavy duty juicer.

The best brands of this type of heavy duty juicing machines make easier the task of cleaning them since the pulp of the fruits and vegetables you use is ejected aside to a compartment within the juicer. A special container is designed to hold all this pulp in the best juicers so you can easily clean it after you are finished juicing. Also this heavy duty machines feature stainless steel blades that make them more efficient and more durable than the average commonly used juicers. Another key feature of this type of machine is that they are capable to extract the most amount of juice from your fresh vegetables and fruits without breaking up. Here is an example of these types of juicers:

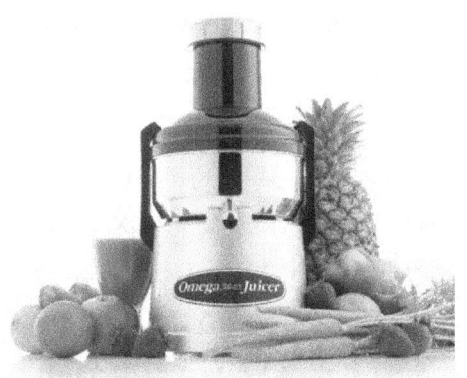
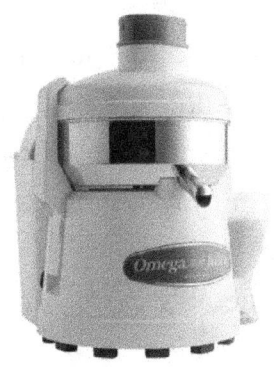

Omega BMJ330   Omega 400 Stainless-Steel

So the ease of cleaning is one essential factor you want to look after if you are serious about juicing. Many other factors have to be considered when trying to pick the right juicer. Of course one of this key factors is how easy is to clean the machine when you have used it. This is one very essential aspect in fact since if you find it difficult to clean your juicing machine you will probably not use it as much as desired. **The best juicers in terms of ease of cleaning are those that feature removable parts that can be washed using your dishwasher so it is practical to use it and be maintained**.

Another key factor that you may want to consider is that your juice extractor is not so heavy so you can handle it without any problems. Also it is an advantage to have a juicer that it is not too big so you don´t have problems with its storage although some juicers can have a fixed place assigned in your kitchen if you juice frequently. These machines are usually beautifully designed appliances that decorate your kitchen with grace. If you are passionate about juicing you also may want to consider an extractor with a wide mouth so you can feed all the fresh fruits and vegetables you want without having any problems. **This will save you time since you won't have to chop your veggies and fruits into small pieces before juicing them**.

An additional aspect you should be looking for is that your juicing machine doesn´t overheat with the friction caused by its moving parts. **Overheating can really be a problem since this can damage the healthy powers and nutrients of your juices**. It is essential that enzymes, micronutrients, vitamins, anti-oxidants and minerals remain intact so you get all the benefits that a healthy juice diet is supposed to deliver to your system.

One tip you can use when you see your machine is shaking because of an overload of fruits or vegetables or clogging is to save a piece of carrot so you can feed the blades and unlock the machinery. But this shouldn´t be happening with a heavy duty strong juicer anyways. **Another important element to be looking after is that your juicer isn´t too noisy,** this can be an indication that the motor is working over its capacity, the best extractors have a low noise factor.

A good heavy duty machine should have a good long lasting warranty on its moving parts and motor so you have peace of mind. This usually doesn´t happen with cheaper models that just offer a limited short term warranty and are not designed to handle a daily usage. In these more economical models the motor is not likely to last as much as with the professional models when put to the test of a regular daily use.

So quality and durability is an important factor to take into consideration when it comes to making your choice for a robust juicer if your idea is to really stick with a healthy juicing diet. Consider this as an investment in your health.

So just to recap here is a list of the main factors you should be taking into consideration when thinking of investing in a juicing machine:

- Ease of cleaning
- How durable it is (quality)
- How heavy it is
- How efficient is the juicing speed
- Is it too noisy?
- What is the usage you will be giving to your juicing machine

So once you resolved these matters it is time to make a decision on which juicer to pick. Here are the different types of juicing machines you can find on the market:

- **The Masticating juice extractor**

This machine reduces foam production. You get thicker pulpy juices with this type of juicer. So it is a great machine to have if you are also thinking of giving it other uses like making baby food, thicker smoothies, ice creams and even healthy sauces. Its mechanism masticates the product you feed prior to a grating process handled by its blades and extracts the juice from veggies and fruits keeping most of the pulp. **With these types of machines you can also determine the thickness of your final product**. This type of machine also produces less heat.

These machines are also referred as slow speed juicers. They operate at a lower speed than other juicers maintaining more of the nutrients and enzymes that faster machines can. This fact prevents premature oxidation and makes it possible to store your healthy juices for up to 72 hours without degradation. It is a great machine to be used with leafy greens and wheatgrass. This machine is basically a strong type of food processor that can handle almost every type of food like nuts; it can extrude pasta and shred herbs. Here is a great example of one these types of slow speed juicers that I really recommend for its multiple capabilities and very good quality:

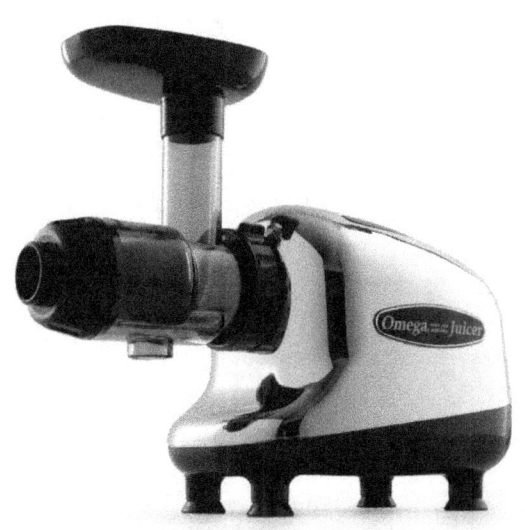

Omega J8005

- Centrifugal Juicer

This is a more affordable type of juicer that is easy to use and also very easy to be cleaned. It just has a spinning blade and less moving parts than a masticating juice extractor machine. Although it is simple it is a very versatile machine where you can also prepare lots of fresh vegetable and fruit juices. A good quality centrifugal juicer like the Breville BBL605XL is an excellent machine that can handle hard and soft ingredients. It has low speed and high speed capabilities and low hit to protect nutrients and enzymes. **This machine can handle big chunks of fruits and vegetables so it is not necessary to chop them previously to be juiced**. This machine also comes with a pulp ejecting feature that collects all the pulp in a separate container and it is easy to clean. It is made from stainless steel making it a very durable and a clean beautiful looking appliance for your kitchen.

Alternative citrus accessories are available for the Omega 4000 and the Omega 1000 juicer so you can squeeze every drop of juice out of your lemons, limes and oranges.

- Triturating Juicers

These types of machines are slower than the majority of juicers and they require a two-step process. During the first step fruits and vegetables are crushed and on the next step the machine presses the juice. **More enzymes, minerals and vitamins are preserved using this type of slow**

juicer. Although this type of <u>triturating juice machine</u> is very slow **the quality of the juices you obtain with it are optimal conserving all its anti-oxidants and healthy powers**. This is a perfect juicer to process leafy greens, carrots, beets, root vegetables, sprouts and wheatgrass.

How do Blenders Differentiate from Juicing Machines:

Basically the most important difference is on the product you obtain using one or the other. With blenders the fiber isn´t separated from the fruit or the veggies compared with juicing machines that in fact do really isolated the fiber from the obtained juice. **When you put fresh fruits and vegetables into a blender machine everything that is contained inside the blender container remains within the end result.** This includes the fiber and any added water that you used to mix your ingredients. This machine features high speed rotating blades that shreds and cuts into very small pieces whatever you put inside.

This type of device is ideal for preparing smoothies where you can mix many type of ingredients like yogurt, milk, ice and fresh fruits and vegetables. Of course for the purpose of detox no dairy products are recommended. When mixed together in a blender all the fiber is retained including flesh, seeds, and the fruits or vegetable peel.

If you decide to use a blender for juicing one with a powerful motor and strong blades is what I recommend you so it can handles different types of ingredients and can crush the ice if you want to make some smoothies. If you want to separate the fiber to obtain only the juice you can use a strainer and the amount of water you put in the mix is entirely determined on how thick or thin you like your juices.

Juices that are prepared this way should be consumed ideally immediately just after mixing them in your blender since oxidation accelerates due to the high speed shredding that occurs inside the container. The best blenders are the ones with a glass container like the Breville BBL605XL. This is a beautiful machine that features different speeds; it is lightweight and very durable. In this machine the blades have a unique design that pushes ingredients on the bottom to the top so that they don´t get trapped under the blades like with other lesser quality blenders.

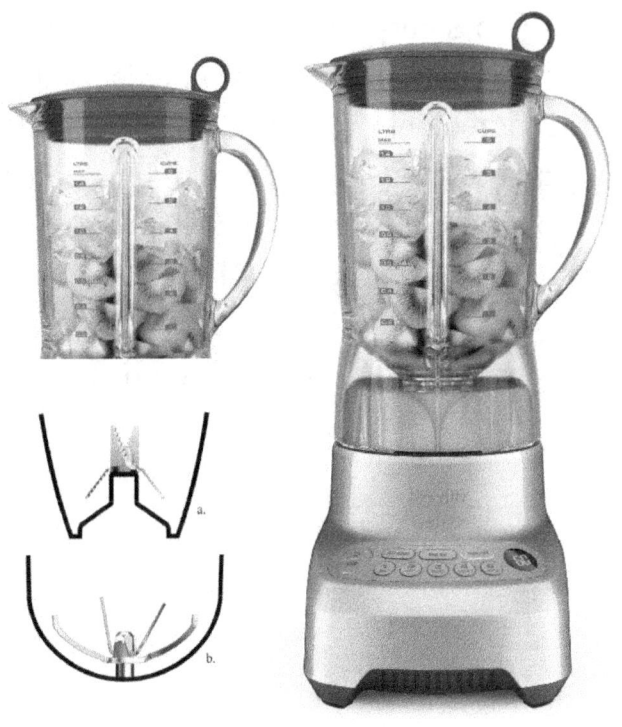

On the contrary a juicer separates the fiber and extracts all the juice contained inside your veggies and your fruits. More nutrients are conserved this way so your body gets the most out of the healthy powers that these natural nourishments provide. **The reason for this is that the juicing process is slower and the oxidation turns out to be also slower**. Another essential factor here is that the assimilation of nutrients and enzymes by your body is made faster with the type of product obtained with these juicers since your digestive system doesn't have to process the fiber.

But for weight loss purposes the dietary fiber kept inside the natural juice is ideal when a blender is used. A blender liquefies the ingredients keeping the fiber whereas a juicing machine extracts the pure liquid making it easier to absorb by your body. Each machine has its benefits but I would say that it is all a matter of how much money you want to spend and how serious you are about sticking with juicing for your health. Anyways it is money well invested.

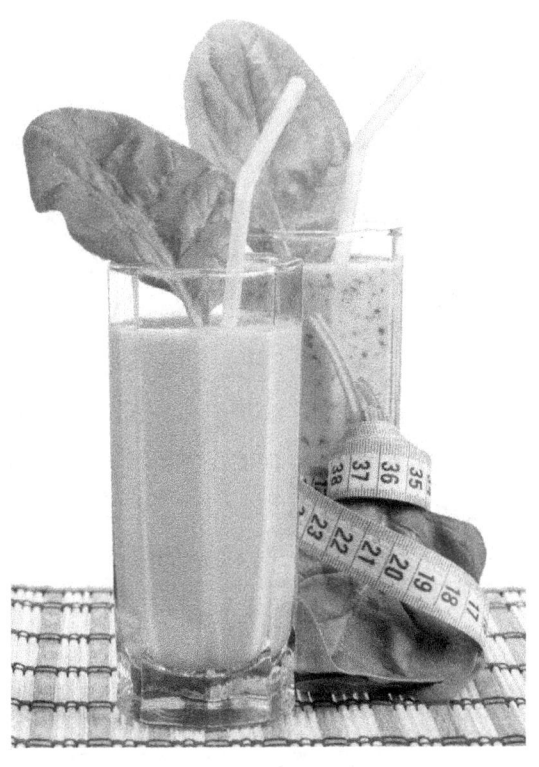

Healthier and Faster Weight Loss with Green Juices

When you detox your body with green juices you not only purify your liver, revitalize your body and cleanse your entire system but **you also get a healthier and faster weight loss as an added result**. The beauty of drinking all these natural green juices is that you get rid of toxins that are trapped inside your body and inside your colon walls. In fact during a green juice fasting period of seven days you can lose as much as 10 pounds of accumulated toxic material that exists inside your body in the form of feces trapped within your colon.

Fasting with natural juices is by far one of the best and safest methods to dump unwanted weight while cleansing your insides. You can stick with a liquid diet for a short period of time like say two days and you will still see positive results. The longer you stay on a non-solid diet based on just healthy green juices the faster and the more notorious those results will be. In fact 25 to 40 pounds can be lost during a 30 day juice fast.

Although it is not recommendable that you follow such a drastic path unless you are really overweight. You can alternate some solid foods during this period if your goal is to lose as much weight as you can in a shorter period of time. But one you followed the initial 7 days detox plan described in this book you will see some very positive results in terms of lost unwanted weight and healthy detoxification. Remember to return slowly to solid food consumption after finishing with it.

A prolonged juice fast is also a way to heal your body from severe intoxication and even to cure chronic illnesses. You can add some soy protein powder to your green juice recipes if you decide to go with longer liquid diet fasting periods to lose weight faster. This can substitute the carbs in your diet and helps to keep your cholesterol levels under control. By adding this ingredient you increase the feeling of fullness so it is easier to go on with your fasting diet.

There are different types protein powders for weight loss but the ones you want to consider are those with less calories, no gluten and no sweeteners and preferably organic. I don´t recommend adding this ingredient to your healthy green juices unless you plan to stick with your fasting for a period longer than 7 days. I you do so just add a tablespoon to the mix only once or twice a day.

32 to 65 ounces of green juice every day approximately is more or less what you need to get all the nutrients your system requires while detoxifying and losing weight at the same time. Another healthy extra that you can add to your juice recipes are organic flax seeds for extra fiber and protein. This ingredient also has a great natural taste that gives you juices a nutty flavor. **Adding this healthy ingredient is great for constipation and for faster weight loss**. A tablespoon of organic flax seeds with your juice recipes will do the magic.

One of the greatest things about juicing is that it can be used as healthy wonderful meal replacement at any time. So you can perform an intermittent fasting type of diet where you can replace one or more meals with one of these healthy liquid potions and lose weight faster. Your juice fasting doesn't have to be so strict after you´ve gotten your first pounds out of your system. In fact it is a great idea to stick with your natural juices and alternate with a healthy solid diet from there on to maintain a healthy weight and a slim figure.

Another advantage of juicing is that you can implement this weight loss strategy for just one day or more days and see results very fast. You won´t be putting your health in jeopardy since your body will be getting all the micronutrients and vitamins it need in the form of liquid and with faster absorption. **The added benefits of such wonderful strategy for weight loss are its anti-aging powers and its powerful energizing properties**.

Fasting is an excellent way to give our bodies a much needed rest from toxins and it helps to regenerate our bodies in a positive way, with green juices you get a healthier and faster weight loss. **In fact you will not only**

feel lighter physically but mentally with a green juice detox diet.

Anxiety and depression are often times also associated with an intoxicated body this is why it is so important to return to what nature has given us and what a better way to enjoy it than in the form of healthy natural green juices.

Let your recovery process start right now! In fact everybody should devote a period of time to a healthy fasting diet based on natural green juices. The results for our overall health are just too amazing to be ignored and we owe it to our bodies to give them a much needed rest and care curing illnesses without the use of prescription drugs.

Discover the Amount of Fiber
Contained in Fruits and Vegetables

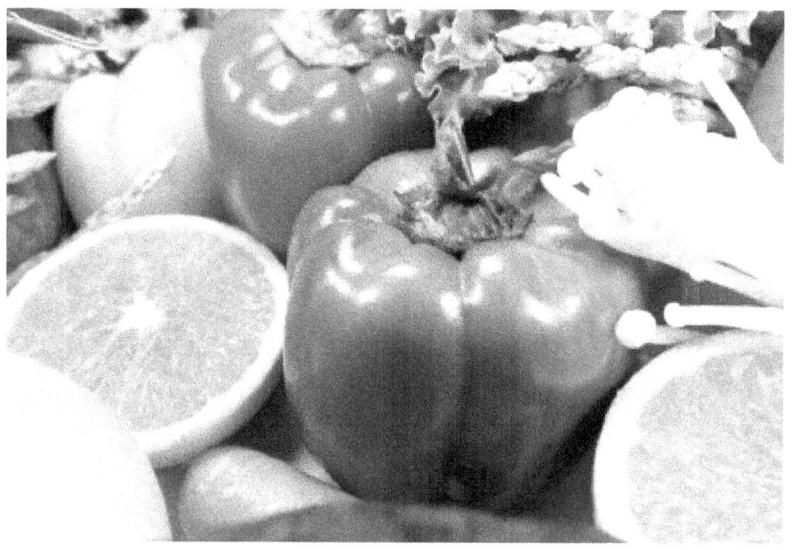

Here is a list of the amount of fiber contained in most
vegetables and fruits that will serve you as a useful guide
when trying to choose the right ingredients for your
healthy menus from now on to maintain a healthy body
and a slim figure.

Fresh & Dried Fruit	Serving Size	Amount of Fiber (g) Approx.
Apples with skin	1 medium	5.0
Apricot	3 medium	1.0
Apricots, dried	4 pieces	2.7
Banana	1 medium	3.5
Blueberries	1 cup	4.1
Cantaloupe, cubes	1 cup	1.5
Figs, dried	2 medium	3.5
Grapefruit	1/2 medium	3.0
Orange, navel	1 medium	3.3
Peach	1 medium	2.0
Peaches, dried	3 pieces	3.3
Pear	1 medium	5.2
Plum	1 medium	1.3
Raisins	1.5 oz box	1.5
Raspberries	1 cup	6.3
Strawberries	1 cup	4.3

Vegetables	Serving Size	Fiber (g)
Avocado (fruit)	1 medium	11.8
Beets, cooked	1 cup	2.8
Beet greens	1 cup	4.2
Bok choy, cooked	1 cup	2.8
Broccoli, cooked	1 cup	4.5
Brussels sprouts, cooked	1 cup	3.6
Cabbage, cooked	1 cup	4.2
Carrot	1 medium	2.6
Carrot, cooked	1 cup	5.2
Cauliflower, cooked	1 cup	3.4
Cole slaw	1 cup	4.0

Collard greens, cooked	1 cup	2.6
Corn, sweet	1 cup	4.6
Green beans	1 cup	4.0
Celery	1 stalk	1.1
Kale, cooked	1 cup	7.2
Onions, raw	1 cup	2.9
Peas, cooked	1 cup	8.8
Peppers, sweet	1 cup	2.6
Potato, baked w/ skin	1 medium	4.8
Spinach, cooked	1 cup	4.3
Summer squash, cooked	1 cup	2.5
Sweet potato, cooked	1 medium	4.9
Swiss chard, cooked	1 cup	3.7
Tomato	1 medium	1.0
Winter squash, cooked	1 cup	6.2
Zucchini, cooked	1 cup	2.6

The ideal amount of daily fiber consumption should be **between 30 to 40** grams from fiber rich foods or you can get it with the help of fiber supplements. It is better to consume your vegetables in a raw form or if you are cooking them it is better to use a good vegetable steamer so they don´t lose their nutritional value.

Conclusion

The health of your body is in your hands and we have to be responsible and conscious about how we feed ourselves. Green juicing is definitely an amazing powerful and effective way that serves as an excellent natural tool to eliminate toxins from our systems. **You can implement this type of green liquid diet anytime you feel your body is battered and weak.** The purpose of adopting a liquid healthy diet like this one should be to make a dramatic change in your eating habits and turn to a more naturally oriented nutrition from there on. **Your body deserves to be treated right and not to be abused with unhealthy foods like processed foods and excess fats.** I want to congratulate you for taking the steps for a better and healthier you and I truly hope that the recipes in this book will make a positive difference and a progressive change in your overall health.

Thank you for reading this book and have a healthy lifestyle now!

Please let me know if you liked this book by leaving a positive review here:

http://tinyurl.com/green-drink-review

Get your FREE Green Tea Benefits Report here:
http://tinyurl.com/green-tea-report

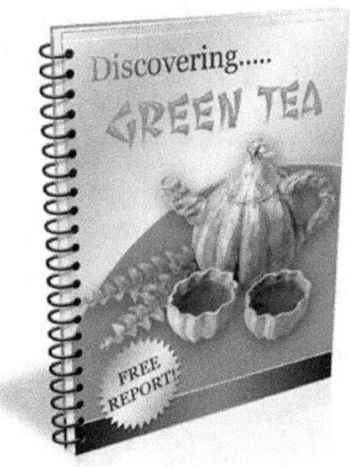

Other Titles You May Like:

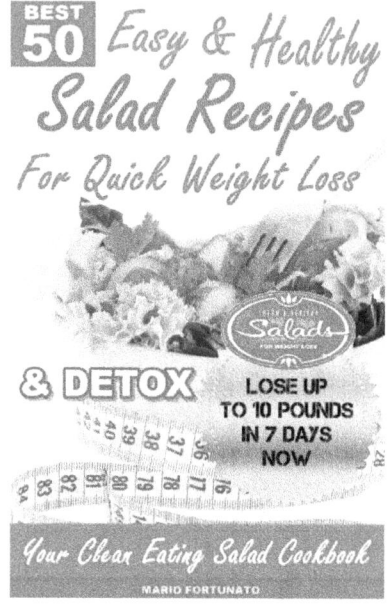

http://tinyurl.com/easy-healthy-salads

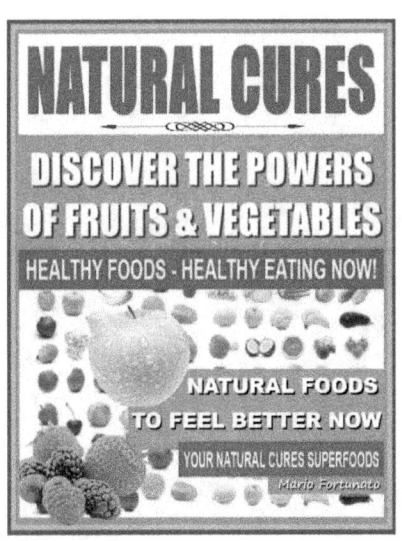

http://tinyurl.com/natural-cures-now

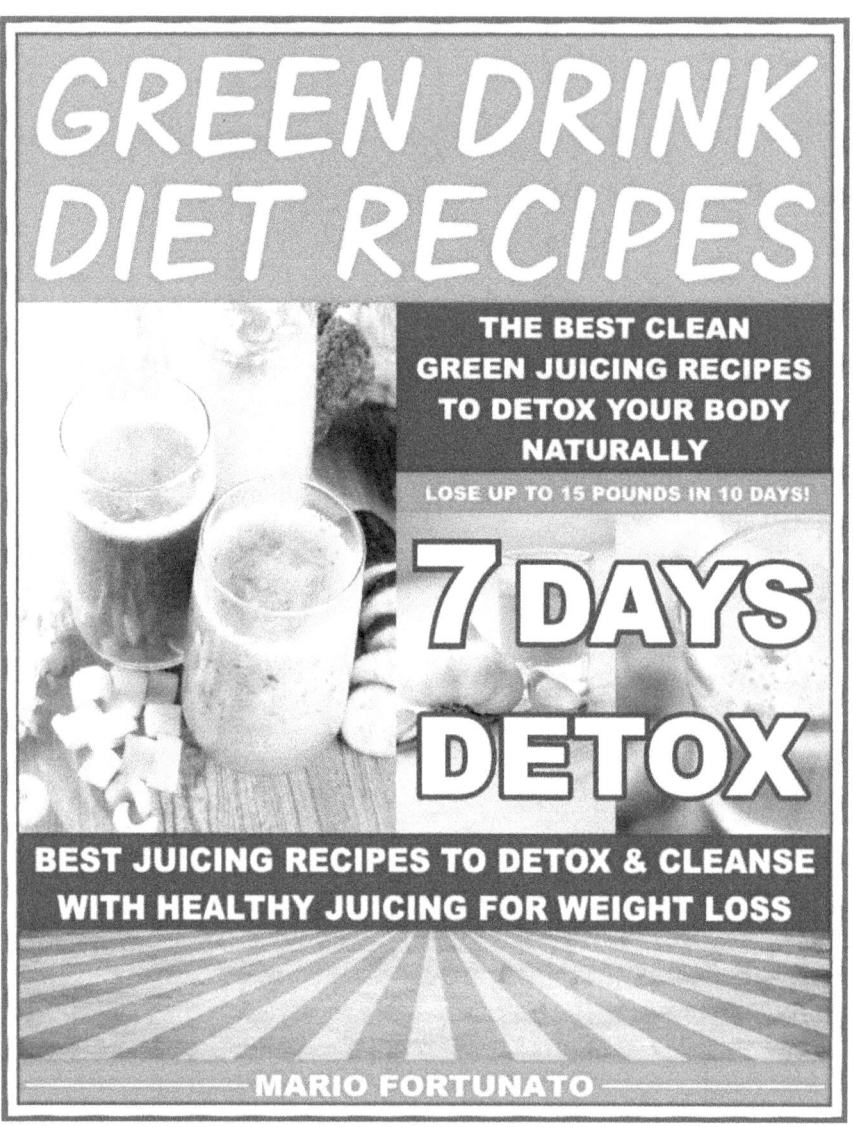

www.ingramcontent.com/pod-product-compliance
Lightning Source LLC
Chambersburg PA
CBHW070538290526
45790CB00002B/545